Date Due

AIDS

AIDS TO INDEPENDENCE
A guide to products for the disabled and the elderly

Irene Crawford

SELF-COUNSEL SERIES

International Self-Counsel Press Ltd.
Vancouver   Toronto

Self-Counsel Press Inc.
Seattle

Printed in Canada

Printed in Canada

First edition: May, 1985

Cataloguing in Publication Data

Crawford, Irene, 1927-
   Aids to Independence

(Self-Counsel series)
ISBN 0-88908-608-7

1. Self-help devices for the disabled.
2. Aged - Care and hygiene.   I. Title.   II. Series.
HV1568.C72 1985   649.8'028   C85-091007-2

Cover props courtesy of Ammundsen Medical Supply Ltd., 1062 Homer Street, Vancouver, B.C., V6B 2W9

Cover design by Sara Woodwark

SELF-COUNSEL SERIES

International Self-Counsel Press Ltd.
Editorial Office
306 West 25th Street
North Vancouver
British Columbia V7N 2G1
Canada

Self-Counsel Press Inc.
1303 N. Northgate Way
Seattle
Washington, 98133 U.S.A.
(a subsidiary of International Self-Counsel Press Ltd.)

To my husband
Tony
who has always believed in me

CONTENTS

ACKNOWLEDGMENTS

Susanne Derbyshire and Michelle Lemon of Doncaster Medical, London, Ontario

whose assistance has been invaluable.

Steve Levine of Maddak Inc.,
and
Doug Nevard of J. A. Preston Corporation

for their encouragement and assistance in providing photographs.

Please note that not all products illustrated here are necessarily available from the company that provided the photograph — the products may be available from several manufacturers and distributors.

INTRODUCTION

The greatest of all human benefits is that, at least, without which no other benefit can truly be enjoyed — independence.

Parke Goodwin

Although the words independence and dependence are separated by only two letters, they are worlds apart in meaning. Independence is like a tall, straight soldier marching along with dignity and self-esteem, while dependence slumps along like an enemy in retreat, with inferiority and worthlessness as companions.

To bridge this gap, to turn defeat into victory, aids and protheses have been developed to help people help themselves: everything from electric wheelchairs to talking books, from tea kettle holders to curved bath brushes. These are just some of the aids that put within reach the goal for which most people strive —independence.

When affliction strikes, whether it be aging, disease or accident, a new lifestyle has to be developed. Dependence goes against our normal grain. Building a new lifestyle is not easy, but aids can compensate. While they can never replace what has been lost, they can assist in regaining independence.

Aids are now big business. Sometimes they are sold unscrupulously, often to those who can ill-afford them. An aid has to be right for an individual's needs. An aid cannot be purchased because "someone else with a similar disability was helped by this aid." Each person is unique. Each person's need is different.

Aids are of value only if they increase mobility and independence. Too many well-intentioned friends and relatives buy them without considering if they are right for the particular user. Doctors, nurses, therapists, and professionals are best qualified to judge the aid. I cannot stress too strongly that no aid should be bought without proper consultation.

Aids to Independence was written to help senior citizens and the handicapped become, and stay, independent at home. It is a guide to what is on the market and is designed to provide knowledge and assistance to laypeople and professionals alike, pointing out the new inroads that have been made in the field of therapeutic medicine. We are now on the threshold of a new era in microtechnology and computerization. Both can be used in rehabilitative medicine to bridge the chasm between dependence and independence and to translate self-reliance into self-respect.

Many small companies that produce these products are springing up across North America. They are far too numerous to mention, but their value and potential is inestimable. Often these companies work in conjunction with rehabilitation and geriatric facilities. They design, develop, and market aids after endless trials of prototypes. Some names and addresses are in the Appendix.

INTRODUCTION

It is hoped this book will motivate others, professionals and laypeople alike, to find the right aid for each user, regardless of whether that aid is purchased on the commercial market or made at home. The cost is irrelevant; the individual's need is the only requisite.

For those who must develop a new lifestyle, aids can help fulfill the new dream — to enjoy life to the fullest, as independently as possible.

Please note: the prices quoted in this book for some aids may have changed between the time of writing and publication. Updated prices can be obtained by writing to the manufacturers or distributors (see Appendix).

1

COMMUNICATION

Communication is a basic human activity, and when we lose the ability to communicate, the quality of life rapidly deteriorates.

Years ago when an ill person wanted to summon help, he or she would ting a bell or call out. The advent of the telephone and its related technology brought an unprecedented breakthrough in communications.

a. TELEPHONE AIDS

Many telephone companies, with their research resources, have responded to the special needs of seniors and disabled people. Possibly because Alexander Graham Bell, the inventor of the telephone, was so concerned with people who had disabilities (his own wife was deaf) the company that bears his name has followed his example.

Over the years the Bell System has devised many innovative aids, everything from amplified sound to bone-conduction receivers. These and more are outlined in their free booklet *Telephone Services for Special Needs*.

One aid is the **impaired hearing handset**, which allows the volume in the telephone receiver earpiece to be turned up by simply adjusting a wheel in the handset of the telephone. When someone without a hearing impairment is using the telephone, the sound can be turned down to normal.

A more sophisticated aid is the **bone-conduction receiver.** This device enables users with certain types of ear damage, or chronic ear defects, to bypass part of the normal hearing process. The receiver, coupled with an amplifier, transmits sound vibrations through the bone directly to the inner ear.

There are also volume control features that can be externally mounted. They eliminate noises in the room so that reception is greatly improved.

For those with minor hearing problems special bells are available: a loud bell for people who can hear only at higher volume, or a single stroke bell. For those with more advanced hearing loss, a horn type of bell is available. There is even a vibrating bell for the more severely handicapped.

For the totally deaf, there is a visible signal, a small lamp that can be connected so that it flashes when the telephone is ringing. These are frequently on reconditioned teletype machines (TTYs), which enable the deaf to communicate. These machines are usually old units that have become outdated by more advanced technology but are still in good condition. With minor renovations they can be adapted as communication devices for the deaf. TTYs look much like a utility table with a typewriter mounted on the top. If someone sends

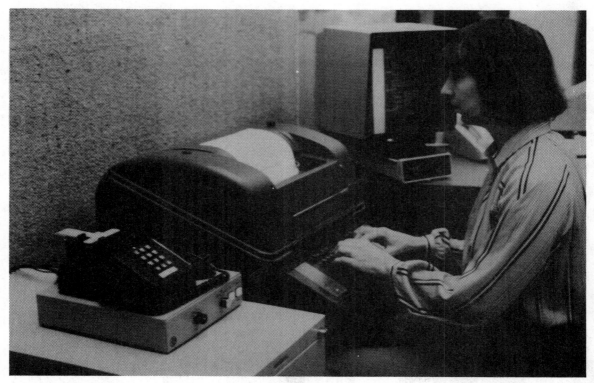

Courtesy of Bell Canada.

TTY — Reconditioned teletype machines for the deaf.

the user a message, the words appear on a print-out just above the typewriter carriage. The user can acknowledge receipt of the message by typing out words of response on the keyboard of the typewriter. Many Telecare and Teleassure or distress centers have the necessary equipment to receive and send messages via TTYs to the deaf.

For people who have trouble speaking, the **telephone amplifier** allows those with weak speech to carry on normal conversations. This, as with the earpiece volume control, is done by adjusting a wheel in the handset.

To help those with an artificial larynx an electronic unit substitutes electronic for natural voice vibrations; sound is produced when the electric larynx is placed against the throat. This artificial larynx is portable and can be used with or without a telephone. It generally makes speech possible.

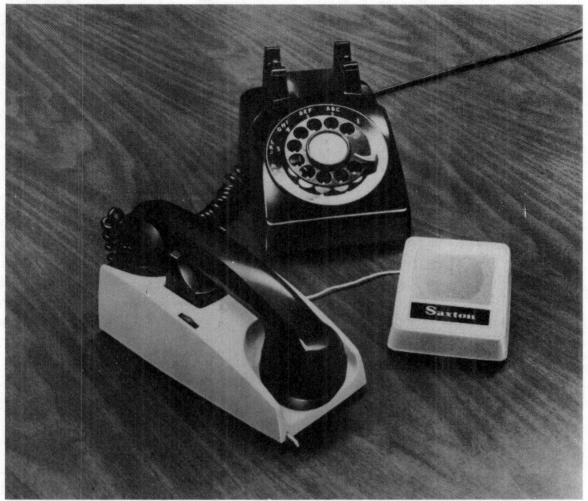

Telephone amplifier.

Courtesy of Maddak Inc.

The **Contempra phone, telephone extension arm,** and **phone holder clip** are devices that make telephoning easier for stroke victims. These aids are usually provided free of charge, except for a minimal installation fee.

Other telephone aids can be purchased separately, such as the **pushbutton adapter,** which is an attachment with large touch tone buttons for those who cannot manage the small buttons. These work only with touch tone telephones. There are, however, larger numbers for dial-face telephones which make dialing much easier.

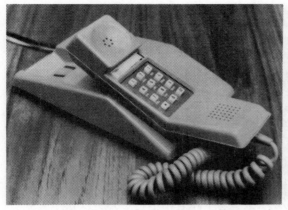

Courtesy of Bell Canada.

Contempra phone — used by person confined to bed. Hang-up simply by pressing button on the handle below buttons.

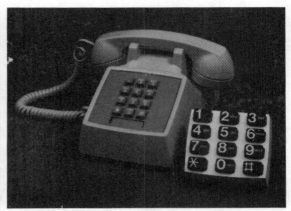

Courtesy of Maddak Inc.

Touch phone attachment.

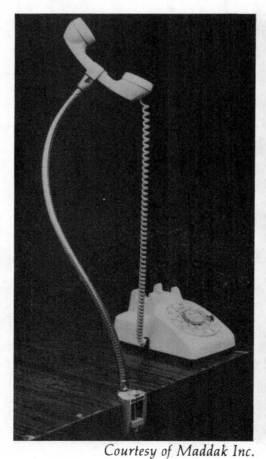

Courtesy of Maddak Inc.

Telephone extension arm.

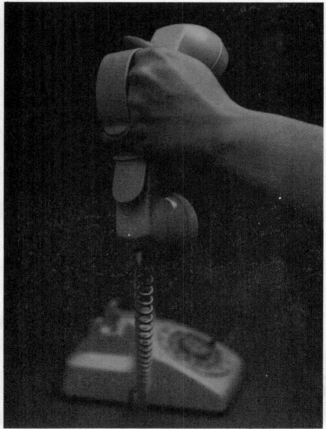

Courtesy of Maddak Inc.

Phone holder hand clip.

b. SAFETY AND SECURITY AIDS

Many seniors and disabled people are concerned for their own safety — both when people are trying to contact them, or when they must call out for help to others.

Since doorbells are a problem for those who cannot hear, a device is available that sets off a flashing light that whirls around the room, drawing attention to the door. It is based on the same principle as the flashing light on TTYs. Most electricians can hook them up for the user.

For those who live alone, many communities have a buddy system where one neighbor checks on another neighbor by telephone. Sometimes organizations get involved, providing a service called **Teleassure, telecare** or **ring-a-day check.** But by whatever name, it assures families and friends that the person living alone is well at that particular time of the day. However, as good as these checks are, they do not cover the time span in between, especially at night when those living alone are most vulnerable.

During the last four years or so, a number of firms have been dabbling in microelectronics, trying to fit modern day technology to the age-old problem of a person trying to communicate if suddenly incapacitated. ProtectAlert, Mircrolert and Medic Alarm are only a few who have entered this field; each have the same basic technical premise involved in their systems.

Although the technology is complex, the concept for the user is simple. While ProtectAlert has a central response center manned by Bell Telephone trained operators, many of the other firms rely on tapes to dial the appropriate sources.

The system consists of a small transmitter about the size of a cigarette package. This waterproof transmitter is either clipped to the user's belt, shirt, blouse or skirt, stuffed in a pocket, or worn as a pendant. The Swiss are currently developing something along this line to be worn as a watch.

The unit base that houses the microelectronic technology for ProtectAlert looks like a bulging briefcase. It hooks into both an electric outlet and a telephone jack on the existing telephone system. This hook-up in no way interferes with the telephone's operation.

To activate the transmitter, a small rectangular button is pressed. With a pendant, the sides are squeezed or clutched. This transmits a signal into the unit base which then takes over. In the ProtectAlert system the signal is transmitted to a central response center, where an operator immediately calls the residence where the distress call originated. This procedure is simply a check for false alerts; sometimes the transmitter is accidentally activated. If there is no answer after three rings, or more if the user is known to have mobility problems, the operator goes to a list of five people who have agreed to accept emergency calls for this particular user. If none of the five can be reached the operator immediately calls the emergency back-up, such as an ambulance or the police. Less than five minutes after the alert signal is received, help should be on the way.

COMMUNICATION

The drawbacks to the system are far less consequential than the potential for peace of mind. Transmitters must be carried at all times, even when showering. They will only work within 200 to 300 feet (61 to 91 metres) of the unit base. They do not yet work on party lines in rural areas.

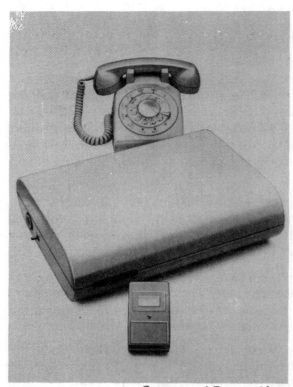

Courtesy of ProtectAlert.

ProtectAlert transmitter and base unit.

Courtesy of United Care Limited.

Call+Care kit.

In the United States, the Veteran's Administration has given their seal of approval to the emergency alarm system. In Canada, pressure is being put on both federal and provincial governments to subsidize this system for senior citizens. In some communities, service clubs are subsidizing the cost. While some of these microelectronic systems can be purchased outright, for senior citizens, rental seems more feasible, as there is less outlay and no long-term commitment. Rentals are about $20 per month, plus a one-time installation fee.

Call+Care is an alarm system from Ireland which recently made its debut on the European market. Now this home-care communication system is beginning to penetrate the North American market. It is designed specifically for the at home patient, although a sister product has been operating in hospitals and nursing homes for several years. Call+Care consists of mainly a weight sensor that is placed under the bed legs, an alarm, and a call button. According to its manufacturer, it is both a sight and sound alarm.

As an alarm, it allows someone in bed to contact a helper by simply pressing the call button. For the incoherent or dementia patient, its weight sensor offers sight to the home attendant by sounding if the patient leaves the bed. Call+Care thus provides instant communication anywhere in the house, relieving stress and strain on all parties concerned, and eliminating the need for constant checking on the patient.

The Call+Care kit comes with cable and batteries. However, transformers are available to run the system on electricity. Another plus for the unit is that it costs nothing to install.

Call+Care is manufactured by United Care Ltd., 7 Lower Fitzwilliam Street, Dublin 2, Ireland, and is distributed in Canada by Medical Mart Supplies of Mississauga, Ontario and C.M. Carpenter Ltd., of Stellarton, Nova Scotia. United States inquiries can be sent to the Irish Export Board, 10 East 53rd Street, New York, N.Y. 10022, or directly to Ireland.

c. INFORMATION AIDS

Coupled with alerts and alarms, there is also the need for the communication of ideas and information, and the channeling of knowledge about products and people, about self-help aids and where to get them.

Accent on Information is the name of a computerized information program developed by *Accent on Living* magazine and Illinois State University. The university's computer has "a convenient listing of products designed to aid the disabled in virtually every phase of living."

The main feature of this program is that Accent on Information "does the legwork, the initial research," and the client does the rest. As a non-profit organization, it has been serving disabled persons, rehab professionals, and seniors for more than 12 years. Accent on Information takes your question about what assistive devices might be available, and the activities of daily living with which you might have a problem, and transfers them to a computer card. This card is then fed into an IBM system where 5,000 pieces of information are stored on data tapes. The data bank is kept current by frequent additions of new products and the removal of those no longer available in the marketplace. It provides a printout which lists special products, books, magazines, and ideas from other people who might answer or solve your problem. If it is an article in a magazine, the printout will tell you about it; if it is a product, the printout will give the manufacturer's name and address, so you can write for more details. Subject areas included are eating, drinking, grooming, handicrafts, mobility aids, legislation, and many more.

The *Accent on Living* magazine is published quarterly by the Cheever Publishing Company, Box 700, Bloomington, Illinois 61701. It also tells about new products, new ideas, new techniques, things to do, and places to go for those who, despite afflictions, want the good life and are determined to have it.

Cheever Publishing also has a *Buyer's Guide* ($10), which lists more than 450 special products for the disabled and has a new dealer section. All contents are updated in each edition.

2

WHEELCHAIRS

a. THE BASIC WHEELCHAIR

For most people, a wheelchair is just a chair that moves. For a user, it is much more; it is an extension of the body, a functional aid, and a supportive part of everyday life. Yet, too often, wheelchairs are purchased in a haphazard manner, with little thought given to the individual's needs.

A wheelchair is a therapeutic device to help a person who has lost mobility, or who has partial mobility, to function again independently. Unfortunately, for some there is the added danger of too prolonged use, and to counter this, a therapeutic rule of the thumb is: A wheelchair is recommended only if it increases mobility and independence, not if it decreases independence. This same rule, of course, applies to all other aids in this book.

Although the word wheelchair did not come into our language until about 1885, chairs with wheels go back centuries. King Philip II of Spain (1527-1598) had a gout chair, which had four wheels, armrests, a reclining back, leg rests, and a mattress of horsehair. With the exception of horsehair, today's models are not that different.

It was the coming of the safety bicycle that really revolutionized the design of wheelchairs. In about 1890, Peter Gendron, the founder of what is believed to be the oldest wheelchair factory in te United States, made the first wheelchair with wire-spoked wheels. But it was mining engineer Herbert A. Everest who, after an accident in 1918 in which he became a paraplegic, turned the wheelchair business on its ear. Everest simply would not accept the awkward, cumbersome wheelchairs of his day. By adapting rubber bicycle wheels to wheelchairs, he made them lighter and easier to maneuver. In 1933, he and mechanical engineer Harry C. Jennings founded the Everest and Jennings Corporation, which is now known around the world. There are plants in West Germany, England, Mexico, Canada; the parent plant is in Los Angeles, California.

Wheelchairs must fit the patient, not the patient fit the wheelchair. Since the user must spend long hours in the wheelchair, it must be comfortable and fit properly. To assure the best possible fit, both patient and wheelchair must be measured.

The patient should sit on an ordinary straight chair with a rigid seat and backrest. The trunk and thighs should form an angle of 100 degrees, knees and ankles about 90 degrees, legs vertical, and if possible soles and heels of shoes flat on the floor. The patient should be fully dressed including braces and protheses.

The seat width of the wheelchair is very important. Since the user's weight must be spread over the widest possible surface, with sufficient clearance on each side to facilitate transfers, the seat should be the width of the patient's hips or thighs, whichever is wider, plus 2 inches (5 cm).

Circulatory difficulties and skin irritations can often occur from sitting so long, so seat depth is important too. Seat depth should be 2 to 3 inches (5 to 7 cm) less than the distance from behind the calf of the leg to the back of the buttocks.

Footrests or footplates vary with shoe size. Since feet have a tendency to slip off improperly sized rests into a drop-foot position, which is very uncomfortable, it is important that the leg length measurements taken from the heel of the foot or shoe under the thigh allow for the adjustment of the footplates which need to have a 2-inch (5 cm) clearance.

The seat height is the distance from the floor to seat platform. If the patient will be using a cushion, this must be taken into consideration. An average polyurethane cushion will compress to one-half its normal size.

The right seat height is necessary for the proper distribution of weight and to attain optimum propulsion. Bedides this, the user's knees shouldn't be so high that they obstruct access to tables or desks. A safe clearance is a minimum of 2 inches (5 cm).

Since the correct posture helps relieve strain and fatigue, the height of the wheelchair arm must be correct. The top of the wheelchair arm should be 1 inch (2.5 cm) higher than the patient's normal arm position.

While the trend today is to have lower backs on wheelchairs, the back height, which must provide the individual with support, will depend a lot on the level of disability. The measurement for the back height should be 4 inches (10 cm) less than the distance from the seat platform to under the extended arm. However, don't forget if the patient uses a cushion, the height of the depressed cushion should be taken into consideration.

The following chart shows the size of standard wheelchairs. If a wheelchair is not available, measurements can be taken from this chart.

DIMENSIONS OF STANDARD WHEELCHAIRS

A guide to selection according to body measurements.

	Imperial	Metric
Overall height:	36 inches	91 cm
Overall length:	40 inches	102 cm
Overall width:	40 inches	102 cm
Width folded:	10 inches	25 cm
Weight:	43 pounds	19.5 kg
Overall width opening:	24 inches	61 cm
Seat width at seat level:	18 inches	46 cm
Arm height from floor:	29.5 inches	75 cm
Width between front uprights	16.5 inches	42 cm
Arm height from seat:	10 inches	25.5 cm
Seat height from floor:	19.5 inches	49.5 cm
Overall height:	29.5 inches	75 cm
Length with fixed footrests:	40.5 inches	103 cm

DIMENSIONS OF WHEELCHAIRS — Continued

		Imperial	Metric
Length with swinging footrests:		41.5 inches	105.5 cm
Footrest extensions:		14.5 to 20.5 inches	37 to 52 cm
Swinging footrest extensions:		15.5 to 21.5 inches	39 to 54.5 cm
Seat upholstered depth —	back:	16 inches	40.5 cm
	seat:	16.5 inches	42 cm

Junior sizes are about 2 inches (5 cm) smaller than standard units. Oversize units are 1.5 to 2 inches (3.8 to 5 cm) larger than standard units, although leg length, back height, arm height, and seat depth are the same.

There are a few points to remember: the width of a standard chair's upholstery is 18 inches (46 cm), but if removable arms are installed, extra width is added to the seat. Points of great strain should be reinforced, including seats, although most chairs are fitted with a reinforced canvas-type seat sling.

A heavy duty chair should be ordered for anyone over 175 pounds (80 kg). These chairs usually have a 36-spoke wheel instead of the average 28-spoke wheel. Remember, though, that larger wheels increase the size and weight of the chair, but only to a minor degree.

A **universal** or **standard wheelchair** is one that can either be wheeled by the user or by someone else. To propel the chair, the user turns the rear wheel with one hand, and to guide it, the user simply pushes against the floor with one foot. Most standard chairs have 8-inch (20 cm) casters and 24-inch (61 cm) rear wheels. While some might have smaller casters (5 inch or 13 cm), the 8-inch (20 cm) swivel type are better.

Brakes are a necessity. They help the user stabilize the wheels when that person gets in or out of the chair; they are essential for security. If a person's reach is limited, an extension is available which clamps over the break lever.

Tires also have to be selected: pneumatic or semi-pneumatic. The pneumatic are much the same as those on a bicycle, but they are made of non-marking gray rubber. They have a pressurized inner tube filled with air that absorbs some of the bumps. While their shock-absorbancy is appreciated, pneumatic tires can become stuck easily.

The semi-pneumatic tires are valveless and puncture-proof. Even though they do not have to be inflated, they have the disadvantage of occasionally splitting. Semi-pneumatics do not last as long as their inflated cousins, another point against them.

Handrims are 2 inches (5 cm) in diameter or less, and are attached to the wheel solely for the purpose of propelling the wheelchair forward or backward; it is a drive wheel. For those people who are limited to the use of one hand, there are one-arm drive wheelchairs: the two hand rims are placed on one side, with the outer rim, which is slightly smaller, connected to the wheel on the opposite side.

A hand rim, placed over the rear wheel on the "good" side, also protects hands and helps keep clothing clean or from becoming tangled in the wheel. One minor fault of handrims is that they frequently have too much play.

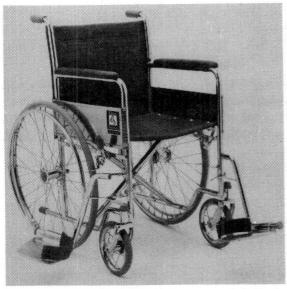

Courtesy of Doncaster Medical.

Universal wheelchair with standard arms and swinging detachable footrests.

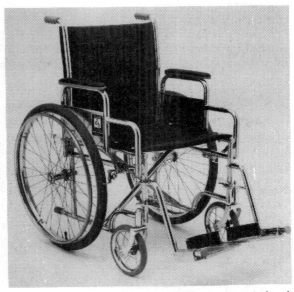

Courtesy of Doncaster Medical.

Premier wheelchair with removable desk arms, semi-pneumatic rear ties, and swinging detachable footrests.

To provide a better friction surface for the hand, a **snap-on-rim cover,** usually made of soft gray rubber, can be purchased to slip over the handrim. Because a wheelchair user often has limited hand and arm mobility or insufficient grasp, handrims can be furnished with projections. These knob projections or spacers, which are ¾ inch (2 cm) to 1¼ inches (3 cm) long, transfer much of the work from the fingers to the palm of the hand.

A more economical way to get a better grip is to wrap the handrim with friction tape. Or the grip can be improved by using gloves with rough palm surfaces. Gloves help protect hands from dirt, friction burns, and calluses, and they protect knuckles from skinning against doorjambs. If a full glove is cumbersome, half-sized gloves that cover only the heel of the hand can be used. Some of these are made of soft leather, but most are made of cloth.

The standard wheelchair comes with a permanent back; however, for those who need the back taken out, there are some equipped with push buttons which can be managed with the use of only one hand.

For anyone with scoliosis, the back should be fitted with tempered foam pads. It is also advisable to have anti-tipping levers on wheelchairs with reclining or semi-reclining backs.

Seats are solid, but should the user need one, a removable seat can be specially ordered. Having a seat that is removable in no way interferes with the other functions of the wheelchair, such as its collapsibility for transportation or storage.

Footrests should be adjusted to the correct angle for the user, so that the knees do not feel as though they are coming up under the user's chin. Also, there should be a 2-inch (5 cm) clearance from the crook or back of the knee to the front edge of the seat. If the seat juts too far forward, circulation to the legs can be hampered. Footrests must also be elevated to a minimum of 2 inches (5 cm) from the floor to allow for clearance.

On swinging, detachable footrests, **heel loops** are standard equipment. However, if a fixed footrest is ordered, a heel loop becomes an accessory and must be ordered separately. Many therapists feel heel loops should be included on all wheelchairs, as they prevent feet from sliding backwards or being bruised by the front casters. For those with weak muscle tone in the ankle and foot, or for spastics, a **toe loop** is recommended.

A **mid-calf strap** is available, but is not considered standard equipment. It helps keep legs and feet in position. **Leg rest pads** can also be ordered for those who need to elevate their legs.

Armrests are adaptable to the needs of the user. Some are detachable, so that mobility is easier both in getting in and out of the chair. Some armrests are shorter and are called **desk arms.** They allow the user to move in closer to or under a table or desk top. For someone who stands upright from the wheelchair, **full arm lengths** are recommended as they are sturdier and handier for someone who shifts to an ordinary chair for eating and working.

b. SPECIALIZED WHEELCHAIRS

Electric wheelchairs have improved tremendously in the last five years. They have progressed from the narrow scooter-types which can be easily maneuvered in the aisles of grocery stores to the new add-on power systems for manual wheelchairs.

Fortress Scientific Ltd., with offices in Ontario, Georgia, and England, have developed an add-on power drive system that can convert an ordinary manual chair to an electrically operated machine.

In a matter of minutes this power system can be installed on most manual wheelchairs. When not required, the power unit can be removed in a matter of seconds.

The system consists of two magnet geared motors with a friction device, batteries, and control unit. The joystick control unit features a high/low change-over switch, battery indicator, horn, on/off switch, and power/manual mode switch. So that the user can come to a smooth stop, a breaking device has been incorporated in the drive motor.

A battery charger for the unit is provided with each kit, which contains two deep cycle batteries; the batteries often must be purchased separately from the add-on power system. The power unit cannot operate during charging, but once the batteries are charged, the charger automatically shuts off. Costs range from $2,000 to $2,300.

Another innovative chair from Fortress Scientific has a power base unit separate from the modular chair or seat. This separate base has small pneumatic tires with pivoting front axles. These smaller tires allow full maneuverability indoors or outdoors.

A special center post design permits the chair module to be mounted or removed in minutes. Most of these modules swivel 180 degrees and lock in a number of angular positions. The seat styles range from recline, traditional sling-type to deluxe models. It is a new concept in wheelchair design. Costs range from $3,970 to $4,500 (including batteries).

A new addition is the Swiss-made *Levo* distributed by the American Stair-Glide Corporation in Grandview, Missouri. This stand-up model with its power lifting mechanism will lift anyone weighing 200 pounds (90 kg) or less up to a standing position. The lifting mechanism is powered by two rechargeable battery packs. The chair itself has handrims, axle adjustments for positioning the height of the seat in relation to the floor, and additional, detachable legs.

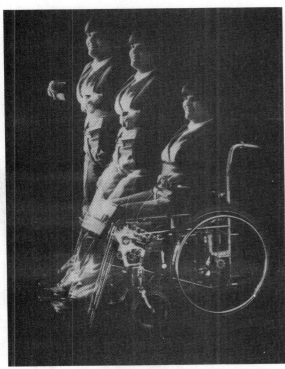

Courtesy of American Stair-Glide Corporation, Grandview, Missouri.

Levo stand-up wheelchair.

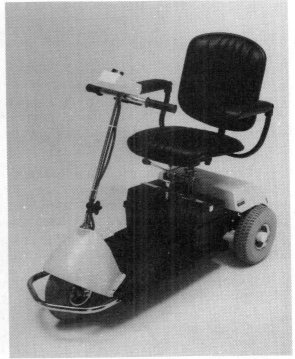

Courtesy of Doncaster Medical.

Fortress Scientific Scooter

The psychological and physical benefits of such a mechanized chair are enormous; users have increased mobility and the circulatory system and other body functions are improved by standing occasionally.

The Canadian Wheelchair Company specializes in the Rogue (a sportschair), prescription and custom-built chairs, and has dealers in the United States, Australia, the Middle East, and the Carribean. Their chairs feature anti-tipping casters. A roll bar is available for those participating in sports; it is attached to the front of the wheelchair and protects the user if the chair rolls over. Recently this company introduced two new models in their Voyager series: the *Active Adult* and the *Active Tall Adult*, which have higher backs.

The electric scooter, which resembles a recreational vehicle more than a wheelchair, provides greater mobility than the traditional wheelchair. The Fortress Scientific Scooter is a prime example.

These scooters are small, compact, battery-powered and easily assembled or disassembled for transportation. They have chair seats, and often feature removable arm and leg rests. All scooters have very sensitive controls, and can be adjusted to fit the user's touch. For example, some units have a seat assembly that can be moved forward or backward to accommodate the height of the user. One model even has a sling seat for hoist transfer. Prices range from $1,500 to $3,000.

c. ACCESSORIES

Many accessories not considered standard equipment can be ordered at additional cost.

Reduce-a-width is a metal device that can be attached to the seat and arm of a wheelchair. By turning the handle, the side of the seat pulls up so that the wheelchair can pass through a narrow doorway, such as those found in many bathrooms. This device reduces the chair width, yet allows the user to remain in the chair.

There are numerous types of **cushions** for both the seat and back of wheelchairs. Because pressure sores are common for those spending long hours sitting, cushions come in many textures, shapes, and thicknesses, from the lightweight, inexpensive foam to the very expensive latex, plastic, and air-cell types. One difficulty with foams is that they have an odor when new, and they also need waterproofing, especially for incontinent patients.

Temper foam has been a big improvement in the cushion market. It flows into the form of impressed shapes, yet fully returns to its original shape even after a 90% compression. Temper foam is a visco-elastic material that reduces fatigue and soreness. It has a firm elastic flow with non-stick properties, and is temperature sensitive: the material gets softer when warm and becomes harder when cooled.

Gel cushions have been available for a long time, and while not too satisfactory at first, they have improved over the years. They are less expensive than some cushions on the market, and allow the user's weight to be spread more evenly over the buttocks. Some gel, and other makes as well, have been designed and manufactured to take a urinal, and these are invaluable to those who have problems in this area.

The **Roho** is a dry flotation curve cushion manufactured by Roho Research and Development Inc., of East St. Louis, Illinois. At a glance, it looks like an inverted egg carton. This rubber cushion took 10 years to develop and is considered by many to be the best on the market for pressure sores. The unit is made up of individual cells; any number of cells can be collapsed to prevent pressure on an affected area.

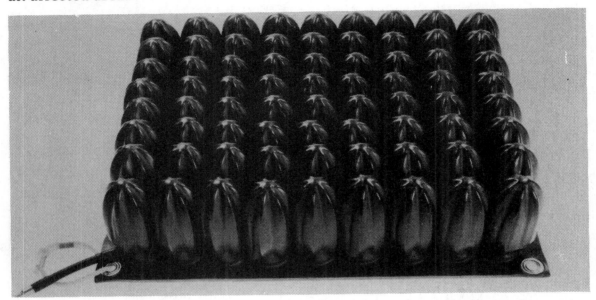

Reprinted by permission of J. A. Preston Corporation.
Flotation curve cushion.

The **jay cushion** is a new cushion on the block. It cradles the buttocks like a pair of helping hands. The unit, which comes in three parts, combines a molded urethane foam non-skid base with a flolite (oil-based liquid) covered by a breathable, washable cover.

Jay cushions weigh about seven pounds (4 kg) and never have to have their fluid replenished. The cost ranges from $129 to $365.

In order to gauge the right pressure, the user simply sits on the cushion with one hand, palm up, under the buttocks. The procedure is to release air by the valve on the side of the cushion until the knuckles touch the seat of the chair. The correct pressure has then been reached. These Roho's can be sponged off by hand or autoclaved. They sell for $300 and up. This dry flotation can also be purchased in mattress size, but with a price tag of over $2,000.

Lumbar cushions are a special posture curve cushion to support the back. They were developed by one of England's foremost orthopedic specialists. They are recommended by the British medical, physiotherapeutic, osteopathic, and chiropractic professions for their help in reducing backache, fatigue, and lower back discomfort.

Skirt guards protect clothing from becoming entangled or soiled in the wheels.

If the person using the wheelchair must also use a cane or crutch, **holders** are available. Some of these holders are straps that fit on the back while others clamp on to the right or left side, depending on the user's preference or need.

Tote bags and pouches for storing items on the wheelchair can be purchased from stores or made at home.

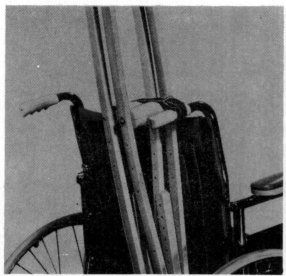

Reprinted by permission of J. A. Preston Corporation.

Wheelchair crutch strap.

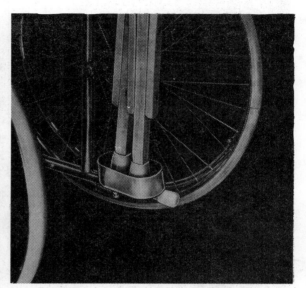

Reprinted by permission of J. A. Preston Corporation.

Wheelchair crutch holder.

Trays for wheelchairs can be expensive. A new, transparent acrylic wheelchair tray has been designed to fit all units. The transparent trays allow users to see their feet, as it is very easy to bump into furniture with the protruding footrests. These trays have a narrow rim around the edge and are attachable with velcro straps. They cost about $75.

Ordinary trays, of course, are less expensive and cost about $25. The most common are made of plywood with a formica surface, and clip on to the wheelchair. These can be easily cleaned with a wet sponge or cloth.

Another clip-on item that is handy for the user and often eliminates the need for a tray is the **glass holder.**

For those who like the outdoors but do not want direct sun, an **umbrella holder** for the back of the chair is available, similar to the cane-crutch holders. For rainy days there are many styles of rainwear for further protection.

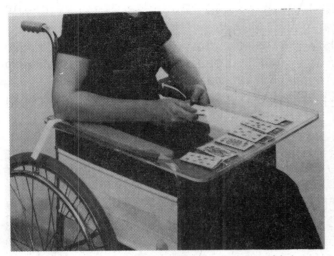

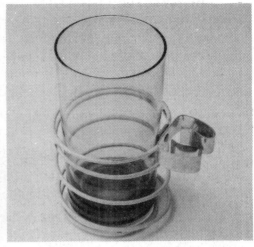

Courtesy of Maddak Inc.

Acrylic tray or lap board.

Courtesy of Maddak Inc.

Clip-on glass holder.

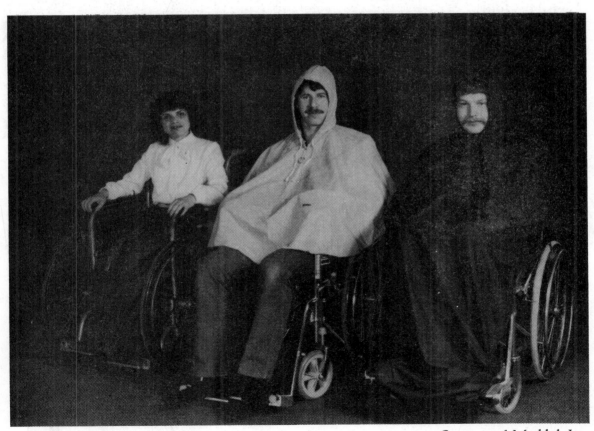

Courtesy of Maddak Inc.

Rainwear.

For those who have cervical limitations or poor peripheral vision, a **bicycle mirror** attached to the wheelchair arm adds depth of vision for maneuverability. For those travelling at night, **bicycle reflectors** or **fluorescent strips** can be attached to the back of the chairs.

d. TRANSPORTING THE WHEELCHAIR

For the transportation of wheelchairs, especially in vans, small aids have been designed to secure wheelchairs when the van is in motion.

One type is made by Ferno-Washington, and provides sunken **wheel cups** for different sizes of wheels and a flush-mounting floor plate with an adjustable clamp operated by a lever. If necessary, this lever will release quickly.

The same manufacturer makes **post cups** to fit into the vehicle floor and hold wheels firmly in place.

e. RENTING WHEELCHAIRS

Because wheelchairs and their accessories are too expensive to buy for a short-term disability, they can be rented by the day, week, month or even year. The rental fee for a basic wheelchair is approximately $35 per week; for one with accessories such as removable arms, the fee runs up to $85. Powered wheelchairs can also be rented, but these run from $120 to the top-of-the-line models at $270 per week. Prices differ by region, though, and are subject to change.

Because the purchase price is so high, it is a good idea to rent a unit for a month, and find out if it is right for the user. If a particular one presents any problems, others can be tried. This way the user is not subject to great expense for a wheelchair until the best model is found.

Wheelchairs are available for rental from such organizations as Red Cross, and in Canada I.O.D.E. (Imperial Order Daughters of the Empire), and lodges that have rental cupboards. Outlets that are often overlooked, however, are nursing homes and homes for the aged, which sometimes have used wheelchairs for sale. People coming to these institutions often have wheelchairs of their own. When they die or are transferred to a maximum care wing, wheelchairs are left behind. The home is then told to dispose of them. Usually the money from any sale goes toward the home's recreational facilities for the benefit of all patients. Resident councils may also take charge of the money to look after other benefits for the residents.

However, if renting from a medical supply store, the first month's rental can often be applied to the purchase price. When a user is finished with a chair, providing it is in reasonable condition, it can be sold back to that store or traded for another model.

3

MOBILITY AIDS

While the wheelchair is a supportive therapeutic aid for those who have lost their mobility, other aids are needed to provide additional mobility.

a. STAIRWAYS AND STEPS

Over the years, many inventors and designers have attacked the problem of self-propulsion up stairs. In 1954, a curb-climbing unit was constructed at New York University under the sponsorship of the National Foundation of Infantile Paralysis. It operated with handrims on level ground, and when the user needed to go up or down a curb, two rotary handles were used, like a jack, to lift the wheels.

In 1965, a contest was held by the President's Committee on Employment of the Handicapped in cooperation with the National Inventor's Council of the United States Department of Commerce. This contest offered $5,000 for the best design of a stair-climbing device. However, it did not produce a workable model, so it was held again. This time, out of 500 entries, a Canadian design was selected. It was a battery-powered unit on a caterpillar track, similar in concept to a miniature tank.

In 1981, the International Year of the Disabled, pressure was again brought to bear on the problems of steps and stairways for the handicapped. As a result, many government buildings and institutions have installed curbs, ramps, and stairway lifts.

Ramps come in many forms. Some are concrete, some are wood, and some are portable. Regardless of the type of construction, all ramps should have a non-slip surface such as corrugated rubber or metal matting. There should be a level area of approximately 4 feet (1.2 meters) at both the top and bottom of the ramp, and there should be handrails on both sides.

A good rule of thumb to follow is that for every inch of height, there should be one foot of ramp, so that an eight-inch step needs eight feet of ramp. Remember, too, that steep inclines for people with limited strength are almost impossible to navigate on their own.

Portable ramps are made of aluminum, and look much like a flat-bottomed eavestrough with a lip. When not in use they can be folded up to half their length and carried like a suitcase. Although fairly light themselves they will hold up to 350 pounds (159 kg) of weight. These cost about $225 to $300.

Hoists and lifting devices are also part of the mobility picture. While new and refined in design, the basic principle of "rope and pulley" for lifting goes back centuries. In fact, still in existence in France today, at the Abbey of Mont St. Michel, is a hoist built in 1202 A.D. The load is raised by a rope around a drum and attached to a treadmill turned by a donkey.

Modern hoists and lifts are usually crane-shaped, and consist of a U-shaped base on four rollers or casters and a vertical mast with an extending arm to which a sling, seat or harness of some type is attached. The slings or holding units are raised or lowered like a boom with a hydraulic pump doing the actual work.

Some hoists and lifts are portable while others operate on a track fixed to the ceiling, usually over a bed, toilet or other facility. They are electrically or battery-operated, and can be stored under a bed, in a closet or in a car trunk. However, most portable units are operated by an attendant.

It is important that, before investing in a hoist or lift, a qualified therapist be consulted. These units are expensive, and their use is not suited for everyone's needs. It is also wise to test a unit before purchasing it; most companies have a rental service where the rental fee can be applied against the purchase price if the user decides to buy.

Some points to consider in selecting a hoist or lift include
- Age and ability of user
- Fitness of operator
- Purpose of hoist or lift
- Amount of space to maneuver
- Amount of space for storage when unit is not in use

While many companies manufacture elevators and lifts for institutions and public buildings, only a few specialize in home devices. But this situation is changing rapidly, due to accelerated growth of the senior population. The American Stair-Glide Corporation for instance, manufactures lifts for stairways, porches, baths, and cars.

Porch lifts come in various designs, with the highest lift no more than 8 feet (2.4 meters) tall. Some models look like an open-top box with a front drop panel.

Bath lifts vary in design and price, with some models featuring slings, and others using a hydraulic hoist with a swivel chair attached. These are great for swimming pools.

Slings, too, come in different styles. Hoyer has a two-piece sling with commode seat. Other designs include head supports and web-straps for security.

For those who like to travel, there are **car hoists** or **car lifts.** These are attached either to the roof or the inside front right or left corner of the car. **Rooftop hoists,** although retractable, remain attached to the outside of the car when not in use. When a sling is used, it is lifted counterclockwise through the door to lower the user to the seat.

Stair lifts are available to fit almost any stairway, and some companies even have upholstered chairs to match the decor. Some models have a swivel seat which allows the user to board the lift in a normal sitting position facing away from the stairway, and to swivel around before the chair begins its upward or downward journey.

While the motors for lift chairs are often under the seat, some models have a special hand-held switch to operate the lift. Others have a lever or button attached to the underside or side of the chair arm.

There are several other **mobility chairs** on the market. One is a chrome-plated, steel-frame unit which looks much like an average chrome chair with casters. This has special appeal for negotiating narrow halls and doorways.

One of the most sophisticated mobile units is an **all-terrain vehicle** which can operate on a 40% grade, averages 18 miles per hour (29 km/h), and is run by a battery with a built-in charger. This battery takes eight to twelve hours to recharge, averaging about ten cents a charge, and lasts from one to three years depending on use. For brakes, all-terrain vehicles have three options: hand, foot, or dynamic.

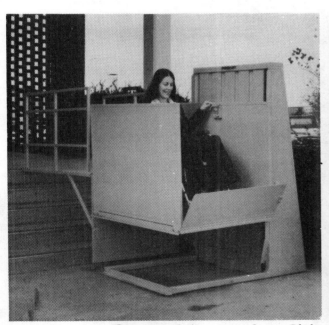

Courtesy of American Stair-Glide Corporation, Grandview, Missouri.

Porch lift.

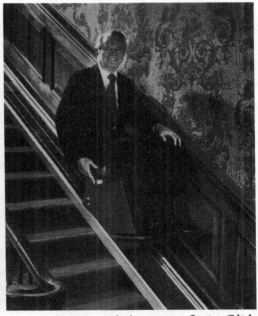

Courtesy of American Stair-Glide Corporation, Grandview, Missouri.

Stair lift.

b. MOBILITY IN POOR WEATHER

People sometimes develop special problems at different seasons of the year. Some are able to get around quite well in warmer weather, but have difficulty breathing when temperatures dip. Joseph A. Nebel of Dolton, Illinois has developed a **personal cold weather breathing aid** which draws warm air trapped around the body into a cellular or honeycomb chest pack. The air funnels up through a flexible hose into a surgical-type mask that covers the mouth and nose.

The mask, made of soft plastic, is held snugly against the chin and cheeks by an adjustable elastic band. This band has an automatic check valve so that the only air inhaled is warm air. Exhaled air leaves the mask through a specially designed one-way valve which prevents cold air from entering.

The chest pack has a series of openings on the side next to the body, allowing body heat to enter and warm the incoming cold air. As this cold air enters the honeycomb pack at the bottom, it mixes with the warmed body air and is then drawn up through the hose as the wearer breathes.

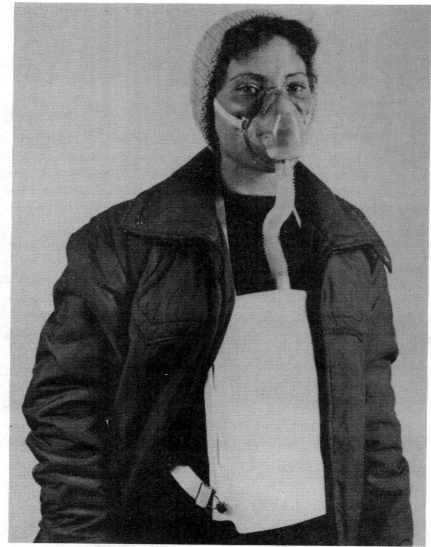

Courtesy of Nebel's Appliances Inc., Breathing Aids, Ltd.

Personal cold weather breathing aid.

The pack is worn inside the outer clothing and does not interfere with vision or body movement. All materials are odorless and are of the type used in hospital respiratory systems.

This personal cold weather breathing aid was originally designed by Nebel for his older sister who had a severe heart condition. Just walking to the car, even when she used a scarf or cloth mask over her face, caused her problems. So Nebel purchased several plastic masks and tubing types, and through trial and error came up with the present breathing device. Further information and prices are available from Breathing Aids Ltd., P.O. Box 62, Dolton, Illinois.

c. MOBILITY IN THE HOME

Just opening a door can be a problem for some people. Arthritic hands, or hands that have lost their muscle tone due to stroke or other disease, have trouble turning a door knob. For them, **levers** are available to fasten directly to the knob to provide easy leverage.

Keys, too, are a problem, mainly because of their size. A key can be inserted into a larger handle, much like the tag often attached to a hotel key. This holder gives the user a better gripping surface.

A new lamp with a touch-on/touch-off base can be found in many mail-order catalogues. A person with mobility or hand problems can simply touch any part of the metal base of the lamp and the light will come on. A second and third touch increases the light, and one more touch turns it off. These touch control lamps have antiqued brass bases with attractive shades. Table models range in price from $90 to $100, and the floor models retail at $150.

There is much to be said for the old-fashioned pull-chain lamp or light fixture wth their loop-finger attachments. Lamp switches are a problem for knotted hands. For those having trouble gripping, a pull-chain with this loop attachment is an aid that can turn a trying task into a simple procedure.

Lamp switch extension levers have been developed to compensate for hand impairment. These extensions consist of a small rectangle with a rod through it which fits over the existing switch. The user pushes up on the rod to turn the light on and pulls down on the rod to turn the light off.

Often, all that is needed to keep a senior or disabled person independent at home is a helping hand. In the United Kingdom, the **pole lamp** has taken on an additional chore other than just lighting; it has become a helping hand. The pole is attached to the floor and ceiling and, instead of lamps protruding from the frame, it has a loop or bar which a person can seize and use to pull himself or herself up to a standing position.

This aluminum column, which is spring-loaded at the ceiling, locks rigidly into place, and the position of the helping loop or bar can also be locked securely in place at any height.

Polecats can be adapted to the needs of North Americans by using existing, but modified, pole lamp frames. However, heavy stress applied from an angle may cause the spring-loader to shift, resulting in both the user and device taking a tumble.

23

Over the past decade or so, **lifting chairs** have become common. Almost any company dealing with therapeutic devices today has developed its own design.

Cardon Rehabilitation Products of Mississauga, Ontario has designed a **geriatric chair** for nursing homes. The chair arm shifts backwards, springing the seat upwards and thereby giving the user that extra bit of assistance needed to stand.

The **cushion lift chair** from American Stair-Glide Corporation in Missouri has stationary arms with a cushion that lifts mechanically. To sit down, a person simply reverses the process. The lifting angle adjusts to the user's needs, with controls on the arms that can be manually or power operated. These chairs come in various colors, styles, and designs, and are the height in sophistication.

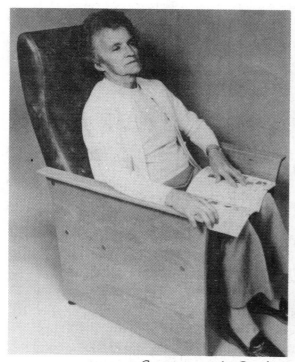

Courtesy of Cardon Rehabilitation Products.

Geriatric chair.

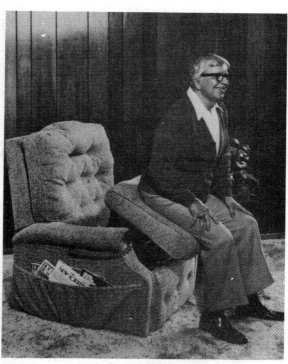

Courtesy of American Stair-Glide Corporation, Grandview, Missouri.

Cushion lift chair.

Gout chairs or **geriatric chairs** were found in France in the early 1600s. They moved on wheels and had reclining backs and leg and arm rests. Today, the backs and seats are upholstered in easy-to-clean, non-porous vinyl. Some have reclining backs and tilted footrests, while others have footrests that extend for comfort and retract for storage.

P.W.L. Inc. (People Working and Learning), a government youth program in Ontario, has developed platform raisers instead of the usual individual furniture leg raisers. Made of birchwood, these box-like stands are large enough for all four legs to fit on the raiser, giving a much sturdier base.

Some people must use a table across the arms of their chair. Such a table has a concealed release mechanism, and, therefore, can be used as a restraint. While many gerontologists frown on restraints for elderly persons, many patients unfortunately do slump down or forward, and restraints of some kind are needed for security.

Restraints come in many forms, two of which are the **vest,** which can be looped around the back of a chair, and **shoulder straps** in the shape of a "Y", which are attached to the chair.

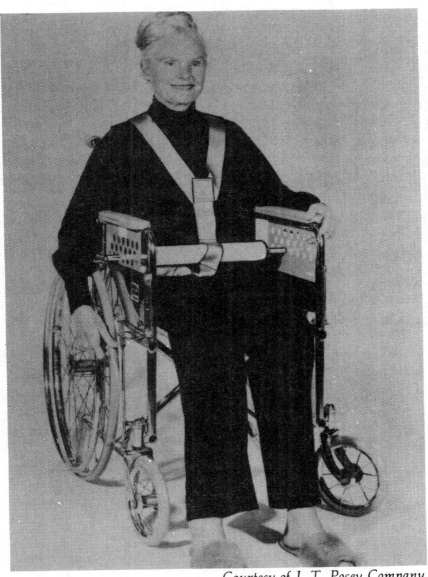

Courtesy of J. T. Posey Company.
Wheelchair restraint.

25

The **safety bar** has been developed by the J. T. Posey Company of California. It looks much like an old-fashioned wooden rolling pin with the handles inserted into a catch mechanism or bracket installed on the sides of the wheelchair or geriatric chair. These safety bars fit across the lower lap and prevent the user from slumping forward or slipping out of the chair, yet they do not have the appearance or the feel of a restraint.

Also on the market are many **flame retardant fabrics,** some of which are used in restraints, from the vest type to the pelvic holder.

d. SYMBOL OF ACCESS

The needs of those with mobility problems have been brought to the attention of the public by a specially designed symbol — the **symbol of access.** Shown as a stick figure sitting in a large wheel, it is used around the world.

The concept of the symbol of access design was first adapted by Rehabilitation International at their 11th World Congress on Rehabilitation of the Disabled in 1969. It is a modification of a design contributed to handicapped people of the world by the Scandinavian Design Students Organization. Its purpose is "to contribute to the protection of human rights of all disabled persons, and especially to an improvement in the availability to disabled persons of the resources and facilities of the communities in which they live."

However, it wasn't until 1974 at Ofir, Portugal, that the Assembly of Rehabilitation International approved and adopted this symbol of access for use throughout the world.

Several resolutions regarding the design were passed at the Assembly: the symbol should always be in sharp contrast, and should be reproduced in either black and white or dark blue and white, unless there are "compelling reasons" for other colors; no change whatsoever in the design should be permitted, and it should be used solely to "identify, mark or show the way to facilities that are accessible to persons whose mobility is restricted by disability;" the symbol of access should always be in the same proportions — an absolute square frame with the stick figure in a wheel; the symbol, which should not be smaller than 4 inches (10 cm) square, can be made of wood, plastic or metal, or of some other rain and weather resistant material and paint.

The symbol of access "represents the hope of independence and mobility to handicapped people" around the world. It can be obtained for a small fee, or sometimes free of charge, at drug and medical outlets and rehabilitation facilities throughout much of the world.

Note that the International Symbol of Access decal only acknowledges that a handicapped person is being transported in the vehicle. The decal alone does not exclude a person from receiving a parking fine. Each person must qualify for eligibility from their local traffic department.

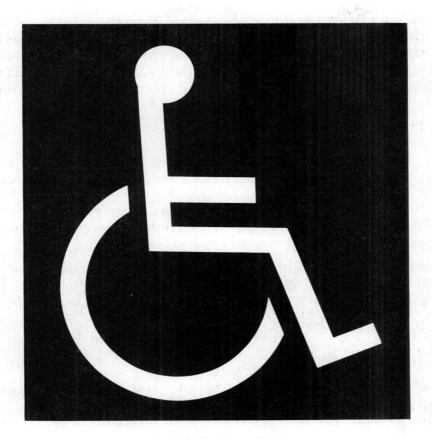

Symbol of access.

4

WALKING AIDS

It was Charles Dickens who said, "The sum of the whole is this, walk and be happy, walk and be healthy."

But there are many people who, for different reasons, can't walk without assistance. Consequently, various aids have been developed to help overcome some of the frustrations that accompany loss of mobility.

a. CANES

Canes are one aid that helps in the drive for independence. They go back centuries, and have had other uses.

In early Greece, they were used as a staff or walking stick, and a crook to herd sheep. In the fifteenth century, they became more elaborate. Many were made out of rare woods and had intricately carved heads. These canes were carried by both men and women for ornamental rather than functional purposes.

By the seventeenth century, canes became status symbols. In fact, they became so fashionable that their owners were subjected to government taxation for the privilege of using them. In England, a petition accompanied by the proper fee had to be submitted to the "Censor," at whose discretion a licence of use was granted. It was not uncommon for young dandies of that day to have their request denied, or have their cane use restricted to certain days of the week.

Men soon became identified by the canes they carried. Doctors carried canes of their own specific design, while lawyers and scribes each had their own particular design. Since canes were an indicator of the bearer's wealth (some men had as many as 40 walking sticks, valued at more than $7,000), more elaborate handles and sticks were designed. Some handles were made of gold encrusted with diamonds while the stick-parts were often made of ivory, glass, or bamboo for summer use. It was a time of elegance but of danger, too. Some men of distinction found that flaunting their wealth brought out the worst of the riff-raff, and before they began to hide long slender daggers or stilettos in their sticks.

Canes are now used primarily to aid walking. The choice of a cane should be determined mainly by the degree of disability, the degree of stability, and the amount of weight it is required to bear.

Styles of canes are as varied as their uses. Some are still made of wood, others are of aluminum alloys; some come singly, others in pairs; some are available from men's clothing stores, others from catalogues. But when a disability is the reason for the purchase of a cane, the cane should be purchased from a medical supply store. Each cane should be chosen to suit the specific needs of the person.

A plain wooden cane costs about $5, while therapeutic models can cost up to $200.

Hospitals, institutions, and medical supply outlets have **adjustable height canes.** These are specifically designed to measure the correct height for the user. Canes should be at a comfortable height, with the handle at about mid-thigh — the body should be in balance, and one shoulder should not be higher than the other or stooped forward.

To adapt a cane to the outdoors, several attachments are currently available. These will fit both canes and crutches. One is a rubber attachment that can be pushed onto the end of the cane. Another is mounted by a simple **screw-clamp.**

Retractable metal **ice grippers** and detachable **ice prongs** in both one and five-prong tips are available to help overcome some of the hazards of slippery walks and ice patches.

All-weather walking sticks with retractable tungsten tips are favored by many walkers. To expose the tip the user simply grasps it and turns the cane clockwise. To retract the tip, the procedure is reversed. Sometimes these tips will corrode, but a few drops of oil over the threads will keep them functional.

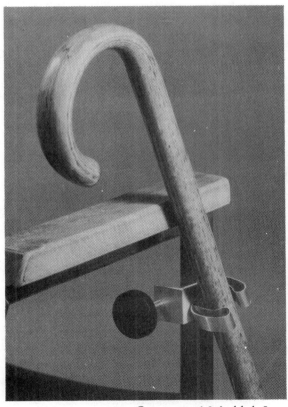

Courtesy of Maddak Inc.

Wooden cane and cane or crutch holder.

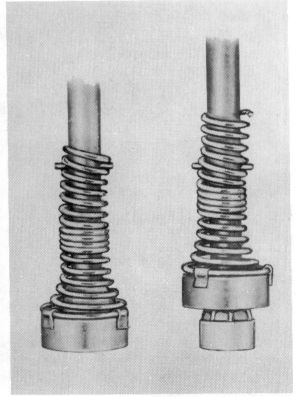

Reprinted by permission of J. A. Preston Corporation.

Ice grippers.

Another cane, much like the hidden dagger type of the seventeenth century, features a hollow center in which, instead of a weapon, five vial flasks for brandy can be inserted. To get at these "life-saving" vials, the user simply turns the handle or pulls off the rubber tip. These are appropriately called **brandy canes.**

To compensate for the various degrees of disability and stability, canes have been manufactured in different shapes and designs. The **offset cane** has a crook on it at about the point where the hip joins the thigh. This design places the user's weight over the center of the cane for maximum balance and control.

The variation of the offset cane comes with a contoured hand grip which will rotate to three different positions.

Walkcanes are a combination of cane and walker. Some styles have a simple curved hand grip with two inverted "U" bars near the top. These are more stable than a cane, yet lighter to manipulate than a walker.

Quad canes have single handles with a four-pronged foot, and have a sturdier base than the traditional stick type. A smaller tripod cane has three steel legs, but these are much smaller and mounted closer to the walking surface.

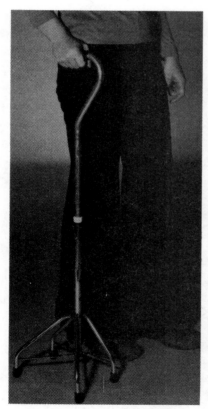

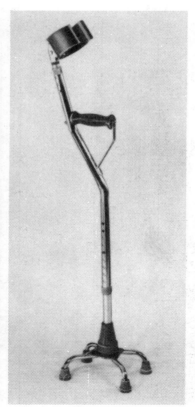

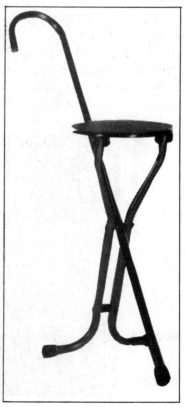

Courtesy of Maddak Inc.

Quad cane.

Reprinted by permission of J. A. Preston Corporation.

Quad crutch-cane for stairs.

Reprinted by permission of J. A. Preston Corporation.

Seat cane.

There are variations of handles on quad canes; some have the traditional curved crook, others have a rubber hand grip, and some have a small rectangular frame at the top for greater security and confidence. Quad legs are also available on offset canes. A stair-climbing quad for an adult sells for about $40 retail.

The **crutch-cane** converts from crutch to cane when the top assembly is removed and replaced with the short handle supplied. The offset design helps to align the user's shoulder, wrist, and tip of the crutch to improve balance and wrist position, and reduce fatigue.

Seat canes are, as the name implies, canes with seats. The user can sit down to rest for a few moments, regardless of where he or she is.

For those who have a little difficulty maintaining their grasp, **wrist straps** are available commercially or they can be fashioned at home.

b. CRUTCHES

Just as it is important for canes to be the right length, **crutches,** too, must be properly fitted. If they are too long, they can apply pressure to nerves or compress blood vessels under the arms. And if they are too short, they have a tendency to slip.

The weight should be taken mainly on the hands, and only slightly on the armpits. There should be approximately a 1½-inch (3.8 cm) clearance between the armpit and the top of the crutch, with the underarm section pressed against the ribs, propping the body on either side. The hand clasps of the crutches should be positioned so that the elbows are only slightly bent with the deflection at approximately a 10 degree angle.

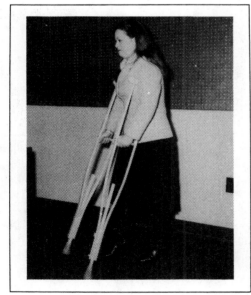

Courtesy of Doncaster Medical.

Properly fitted crutches.

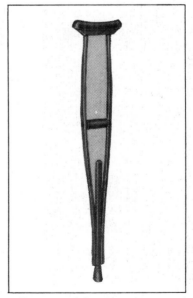

Reprinted by permission of J. A. Preston Corporation.

Wooden crutch.

MEASURING CHART

PATIENT SIZE		CRUTCH SIZE	
Inches	Centimeters	Inches	Centimeters
82	208	65	165
80	203	64	163
78	198	62	157
76	193	60	152
74	188	58	147
72	183	56	142
70	178	54	137
68	173	52	132
66	168	50	127
64	163	48	122
62	157	46	117
60	152	44	112
58	147	42	107
56	142	40	102
54	137	38	97
52	132	36	91
50	127	34	86
48	122	32	81
46	117	30	76
44	112	28	71
42	107	26	66
40	102	25	64

Placement position of crutches

45°

6"
15 cm

TOE OF
CRUTCH

Charts courtesy of Doncaster Medical.

The traditional models of crutches are still made of wood, usually hard maple veneer, and are cheaper to purchase than their more sophisticated lightweight cousins. These wooden models have wing nuts in the frame to allow for easier height and grip adjustments.

Many of the aluminum alloy crutches have forearm supports for using the strength of the arms, while still giving extra support to the hands.

Other items, such as crutch tips and hand grips can be purchased separately and range in price from $3 up.

c. WALKERS

For people who have a problem bearing their weight, or who have a general stability problem, **walkers** provide the extra assurance they need to give them greater mobility.

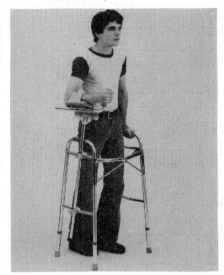

Reprinted by permission of J. A. Preston Corporation.

Arthritic cane-crutch with forearm walker attachment.

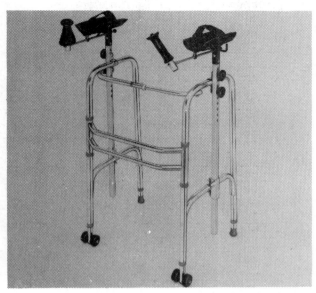

Courtesy of Lumex Inc.

Walker with front casters.

Most walkers are made of aluminum and are designed with a walk-in frame. Instead of handles, they have side and front grip bars. Forearm attachments, which are an added feature, can be attached to the frame if the user has grip problems.

Walkers come in various sizes for children, teens, and adults. Heights are adjustable, and just as in canes and crutches, the proper height for the user is important. Some walkers, to provide greater mobility, have casters on the front with automatic pressure brakes. Certain models have been developed to allow the user toilet comfort, and the frames have been contoured with this in mind.

Plain models range in price from $50 to $150 depending on attachments and adjustments needed.

Rollators and mobilizers have the features of a walker with wheels, combined with the compactness of a fold-up walker. Many have been designed for sufferers of arthritis, polio, cerebral palsy, and related diseases that create walking problems. They are rigid in use, but can be folded up. If the user fails to keep pace with the walker, the rear crutch tips will grip the ground, stopping the walker and permitting the user to catch up. One sophisticated model has a stand support, much like a narrow, padded table top. All units are adjustable in height.

Additional items that can be purchased to supplement the function of the walker include the extension bracket with **handgrip** and **walker bag, caddy or catch-all.**

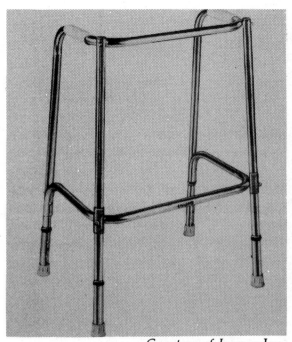

Courtesy of Lumex Inc.

Standard walker.

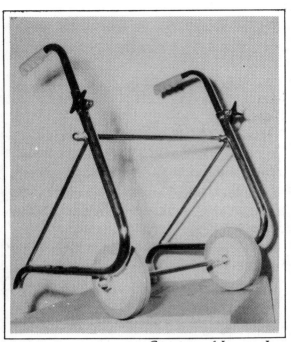

Courtesy of Lumex Inc.

Rollator.

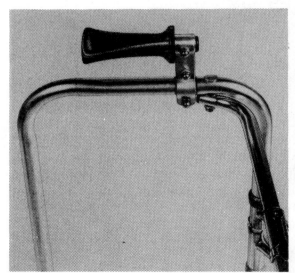

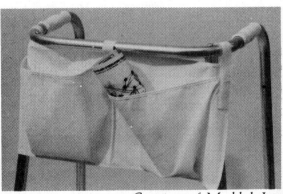

Courtesy of Maddak Inc.

Walker and wheelchair bag.

Courtesy of Lumex Inc.

Extension brackets with handgrips.

Caddy or catch-all.

Courtesy of Maddak Inc.

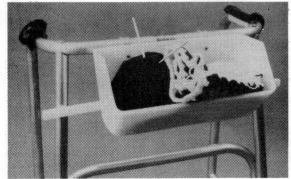

5

COOKING AND CLEANING

Many people, despite their handicaps, like to cook; many others need to cook and clean if they are on their own. Without the help of cooking and cleaning aids, however, many tasks would be impossible to perform.

While some of these aids are quite expensive, a versatile handyperson can adapt the models to his or her needs by using materials at hand.

Reaching sticks or tongs are invaluable in the kitchen. Some have gun-like handles with magnetic trigger mouths that grasp and close. These reaching aids come in various lengths, and some models even fold up so that they can be put in a pocket or pouch. Their use is not restricted to the kitchen; they can be used throughout the house, and in the garden as well.

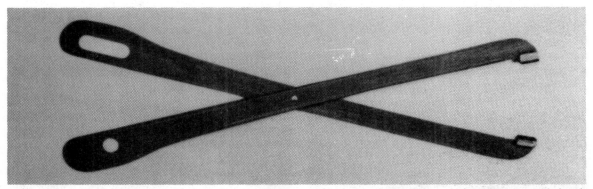

Courtesy of Doncaster Medical.

Tongs.

One reaching aid that can be adapted to various uses in the kitchen is the lowly **coat hanger.** With a magnet attached to the straightened hook end, the hanger can be used to retrieve items dropped on the floor or out of reach in cupboards. The remainder of the hanger can be shaped into a rectangle and held by means of a small clamp, or it can be tightened into a workable handle to provide a better grip.

A strap made of velcro or webbing from a discarded automobile seat belt, for example, can be slipped around an oven door handle. This loop gives the body leverage so that the stress of pulling open the door is decreased for the fingers, hands or wrists. This is useful for those people who have weak muscle tone.

Slide boards are invaluable for people who are no longer able to lift things. These boards are beveled at both ends and have rubber strips underneath to prevent slipping, allowing pots and pans to slide from one place to another without any lifting.

Slide boards can be placed with one end on a portable utility table and the other end on the counter or stove top. In this manner, the utensils can be slipped from the counter to the table, which in turn can be wheeled elsewhere.

They can be easily made from a plain piece of plywood with non-skid strips attached to the bottom. Slide boards also can be purchased from retail outlets.

Cutting boards, which are available at any hardware or department store, can be adapted for those with grasp problems. A plastic edge, or grooved or rounded piece of narrow wood stripping can be attached to two adjacent sides to prevent food from slipping off the board when being cut. Nails or spikes can be driven up through the cutting board to hold the food that is being peeled or cut.

Commercial cutting boards come in various sizes and shapes, and some have removable holders made of nails or prongs. One type of board, developed by the Independent Needs Centre in Willowdale, Ontario is a square block with acrylic extensions along two sides. The corners of these extensions do not quite meet, so there is room for a knife blade to cut through completely whatever food is being prepared.

A **bread slice holder** is a similarly designed device which will hold a slice of bread in place for spreading butter, preserves, and so on.

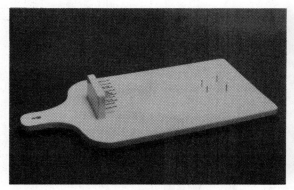

Courtesy of Maddak Inc.

Food cutting board.

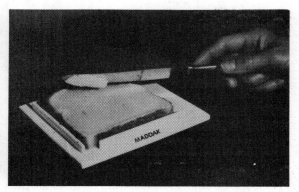

Courtesy of Maddak Inc.

Bread slice holder.

Swivel spoons for stirring are available, although everyday spoons can be built up with foam or adhesive tape to provide a better grip surface.

There is a **one-hand butcher knife** on the commercial market which looks much like the rocker knife that cuts by a rocking rather than a slicing motion.

A cook's knife for those with limited grasp has been imported from Sweden for the North American market. The handle is attached at an angle to a flat-sided blade. These are available from medical supply stores.

There are also many all-purpose knives that can be purchased at most hardware outlets. Usually one or two will have a substantial handle, which is recommended for those people who need the larger area to provide an easier grip.

Many aids found in hardware and kitchen utensil departments can be adapted to other uses. **Marvel brand peelers,** for example, with their wide handles, can be used for slicing and grating. They are of great assistance to users with lost muscle tone. Marvel brands are available from mail order outlets as well, and department store chains stock them for under $3.

Handle holders for pots and pans can be purchased at retail outlets or they can be made at home. They usually have a suction base, and a "U" or "V" upright where the pot handle rests. This holds the pot handle in place, so that when someone is stirring the contents with one hand, the pot doesn't whip round and round with the stirring motion.

Some pot handle holders are just wire frames with small suction cup bases; others are sturdier with wooden bases and wooden upright arms forming a "U" between them.

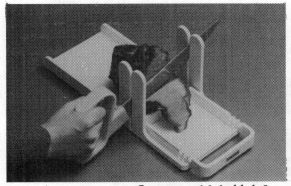

Courtesy of Maddak Inc.

Slicing knife.

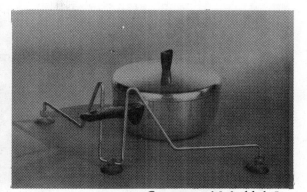

Courtesy of Maddak Inc.

Pan holder.

Strainers are an aid when straining liquid from a pan. These look much like half-lids with dozens of small holes, and are attached to "V" shaped handles which when in use run parallel to the pot handle. These strainers have a spring-loader to hold them securely when pouring.

However, a colander will work just as well, and is a little cheaper. Both are available at utensil counters.

Tea kettles are a problem for anyone who has a problem with lifting. Many aids are ineffective because there are so many different models of tea kettles on the market; an aid that will fit one kettle will not fit another. To combat the overall problem, the Independent Needs Centre has come up with an aid that is not only good for tea kettles, but for other uses as well. They make a box-shaped stand with a heat resistant tilt-top. Around the front and a few inches up each side of the tilt top is a row of pre-drilled holes into which pegs can be fitted or glued. This peg-type fence holds the kettle secure when the top is tilted to pour the water. This same tilt-top also works well for bowls, especially those with spouts.

There is also a special metal frame with a swinging bowl attached. While the bowl is anchored, it still can be tipped so that its contents can be poured into a dish or pan underneath the frame.

Separating an egg might not seem like much of a chore, but try doing it with one hand. **Egg separators** can be bought in hardware and kitchen supply outlets. However, a small funnel works just as well. Crack the egg over the mouth of the funnel, and the yolk will stay in the upper part while the white trickles through the neck into a bowl.

In many large retail outlets, **battery operated flour sifters** and **egg beaters** can be purchased. Both are of great value to people with hand disabilities.

For those who like to bake, a **one-handed rolling pin** has been designed. But again, an ordinary wooden pin can be adapted to one-hand use by attaching a frame. The commercial unit looks much like a paint roller and often comes with a smaller roller at the opposite end for pizza.

Another problem in the kitchen is grating, especially if it must be done with one hand. Some designers have made a **grater** that is perpendicular to a base board and held on the counter top with suction cups. This allows the user to push the food against the stable grater. A similar device can be created at home.

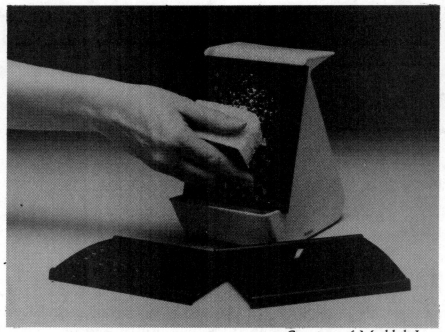

Courtesy of Maddak Inc.

Grater with bin.

Also available from retail outlets is the stay-put grater. It has three interchangeable plastic plates that attach to a bin that catches the grated food. There are several models on the market with plastic instead of metal bins, which have a tendency to rust. However, electric food processors, blenders and beaters have made this area of food preparation less of a problem for the disabled than it once was.

Opening any jar can be a chore if a person is limited to the use of one hand or has reduced muscle tone. There are several **jar openers** on the market. One is the under-shelf type. It is made of durable plastic and can be attached inconspicuously under an upper cupboard edge. The jar lid slips easily into the opener, where it wedges and allows the user to turn the jar with one hand. This type of opener can accommodate any jar screw lid from ⅜ inch to 3-⅜ inches (1 cm to 8.5 cm). However, it will not remove a pry-off cap, which are becoming more common.

Zim is the trade name for a metal jar opener. It mounts on the wall, much like a can opener with its steel teeth doing the grasping. It sells for about $10.

The **belliclamp** is another device that can be used for opening jars, and it has additional uses. This device secures the jar instead of the lid for turning. It rests on the countertop and allows the user to apply pressure to a plastic clamp with the stomach or thigh. This holds the object in place for one-hand manipulation, such as turning a jar lid or polishing shoes.

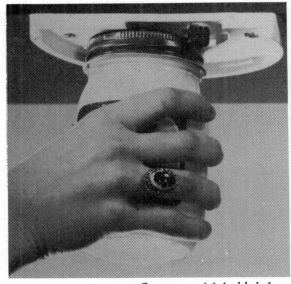

Courtesy of Maddak Inc.

Jar opener.

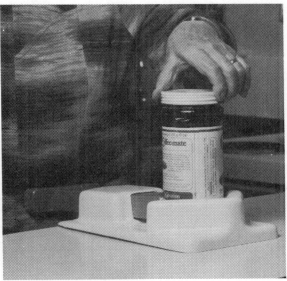

Courtesy of Homecraft Supplies Limited, London, England.

Belliclamp jar opener.

While many **can openers** can be operated with one hand, there are a few models designed specifically for those who have limited grip. A few are available through mail order catalogues.

Zim has also developed a **jar-can opener.** This dual purpose device has a white plastic finish, is wall mounted, and can be folded flat when not in use.

Just being able to cook and bake isn't the whole story, of course; people must wash up afterwards. There are taps to turn, and the sink must be filled with water. Several tap turners are available at retail outlets; one type fits like a hat over the tap, while another type locks on. The contour turner is a tool that aids in operating any rotating knob handle or control.

COOKING AND CLEANING

To help clean glasses, cups or bottles, brushes can be mounted on a wooden base and secured to the bottom or side of a sink with suction cups. The glasses, or whatever, can then be cleaned by rotating them over the brush.

Dishes can always be dried just by leaving them on a draining board.

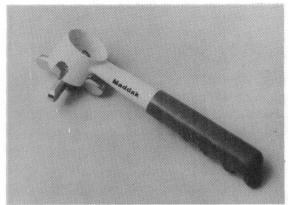

Courtesy of Maddak Inc.

Tap turner.

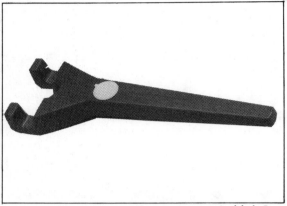

Courtesy of Maddak Inc.

Tap turner.

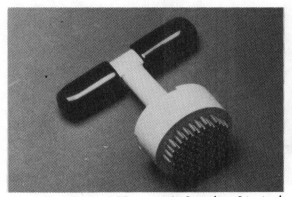

Courtesy of Homecraft Supplies Limited,
London, England.

Contour turning handle.

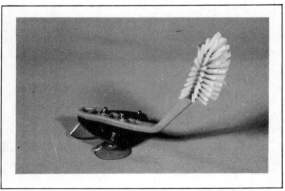

Courtesy of Maddak Inc.

Dish brush.

Sweeping or washing the floor can be a big chore for a person in a wheelchair or someone on crutches. Even someone with mobility, but who can't bend, has great difficulty cleaning a floor. Brooms and dust pans can be purchased with different types and lengths of handles to aid those with problems.

A **self-wringing mop** with a replaceable sponge head is also helpful. The user simply dips the head of the mop into the cleaning solution and pulls the lever to release the correct amount of water. As the user scrubs, foam rubber pads suck up the water. To release the dirty fluid, the user simply pulls the lever again, making sure, of course, the mop is over the bucket. To make this cleaning process easier, casters can be mounted on a board under the pail, or can be secured directly to the receptacle, to provide mobility.

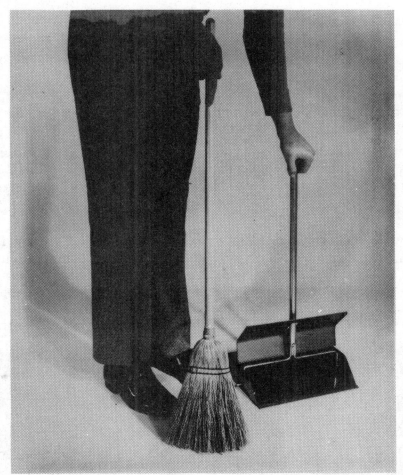

Courtesy of Maddak Inc.

Dust pan and broom.

From our European ancestors, we have the **foot mop.** It is a large, padded, absorbent cloth with a mitt top. The user simply inserts a foot and shuffles over the floor to dust or polish, or mop up spills. It provides the added benefit of exercising muscles, especially in the legs, as one does when skating.

6

EATING

It was the Roman poet Horace who said, "The chief pleasure in eating does not exist in costly seasoning or exquisite flavor, but in yourself."

Being able to feed oneself is a treasure taken for granted until it is lost. But various aids have been developed to assist those who have difficulties in this treasured area of independence.

a. FLATWARE

Built-up handles on flatware are a great asset for those with grip problems. These come with swivel and non-swivel handles, the former having a built-in stop. Other utensils have mouth-end curves, right or left, depending on the need. These are usually made of stainless steel with lock-in handles, but cheaper plastic is available in many instances. These built-in or "bicycle" grip handles come in two sizes, and fit like a sleeve over the regular handle of the utensil.

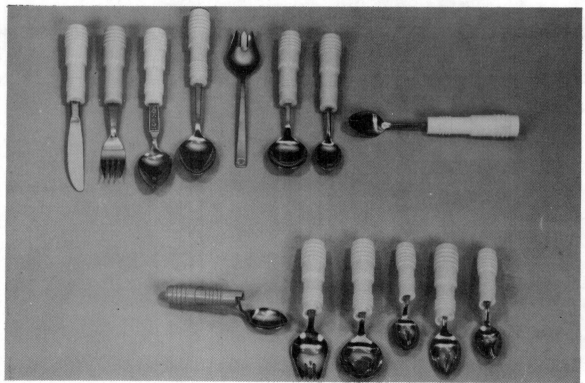

Reprinted by permission of J. A. Preston Corporation.
Bicycle grip handles.

There are angle handles for built-up fork and spoon combination units for either right-handed or left-handed users. People can make their own built-up handles by using closed cell foam.

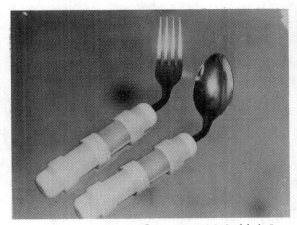

Courtesy of Maddak Inc.

Built-up fork and spoon angle handles.

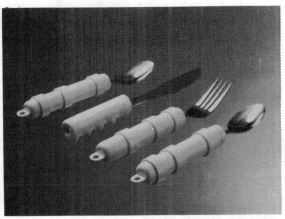

Courtesy of Maddak Inc.

Built-up handles.

Another company has developed a rubazote cushion tubing for building up handles. This tubing comes in 6-foot (1.8 m) lengths with center holes of three different sizes.

The **rocker knife** has been designed for those people who only have the use of one hand. The knife cuts the food in a rocking motion, rather than a slicing one. There is also a rocker knife and fork combination available: the knife has, instead of a pointed end, a three or four-tined fork.

Another utensil, called the miracle or **three-in-one** combines in one functional unit the bowl of a spoon, the tines of a fork, and the blade of a knife. The edges of this unit, while sharp enough to cut food, will not cut the user's mouth.

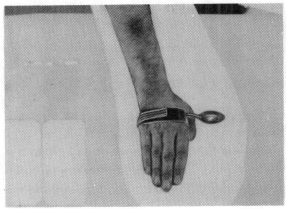

Reprinted by permission of J. A. Preston Corporation.

Utensil holder.

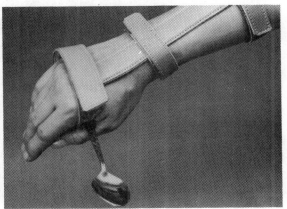

Courtesy of Maddak Inc.

Wrist splint with spoon pocket.

A **rolling knife,** similar in form to a pizza cutter, has a protective shield over the blade. But is has gained only limited acceptance by the disabled and the elderly.

Even with the larger-than-life handles, some people still cannot grasp a utensil, so **holders** have been designed to fit around the hand. Most are made of soft plastic and some have velcro closures, but there are as many variations as there are needs.

b. CUPS AND PLATES

Feeding cups for convalescents have travelled the road with the sick through the centuries. Early designs looked like tea pots, with the spout being used to drink from. Some of these early china models are still in use, with little change in design, although now instead of the full lid, there is a half-opening where liquids are poured. However, the opening nearest the spout is sealed so liquids won't spill.

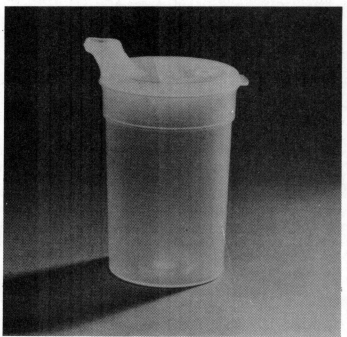

Courtesy of Maddak Inc.

Flow-controlled drinking glass.

Today, the convalescent cup is generally made of plastic, comes in various colors, and is dishwasher safe. Usually, it has a slanted mouthpiece which permits the liquid to flow without dripping when the user drinks. Most cups feature a small hole where a straw can be inserted. Actually there are as many types of cups as there are companies that produce them. There is even a **nose cutout glass** on the market which allows a person to drink without tipping the head back or extending the neck.

No-tip cups have also been developed. They have a solid base in which a glass or flow-easy cup can be set.

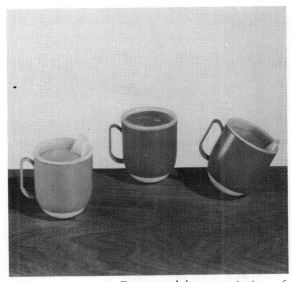

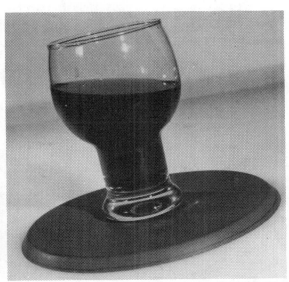

*Reprinted by permission of
J. A. Preston Corporation.*

Spill proof drinking cups.

Courtesy of Maddak Inc.

Non-slip surfaces.

Non-slip bases are available and come in various sizes. Some will clasp around only a cup or glass, while others have a much wider girth and will anchor a large plate or bowl. They can be purchased at most hardware and medical supply stores.

Sectioned plates can make eating a little easier for those with limited hand use. While restaurants have used sophisticated models for some time, ordinary sectioned plates are on the market for seniors and handicapped.

In addition to these dishes, others, called **scoops,** have one vertical side and one sloping side. Some styles have a non-skid rubber pad on the bottom for better control.

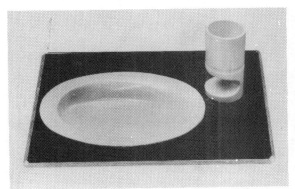

Courtesy of Maddak Inc.

Scoop dishes.

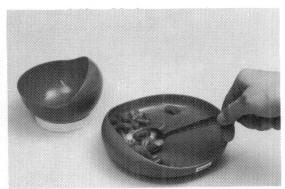

Courtesy of Maddak Inc.

Scooper plate and bowl.

Inner lip plates look much like the old-fashioned wide-rimmed porridge bowls. But like the scoop dishes, they tend to make those who use them uncomfortable.

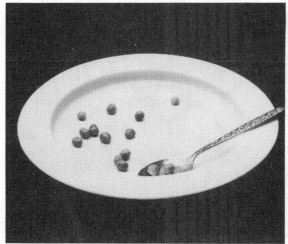

Courtesy of Maddak Inc.

Inner lip plate.

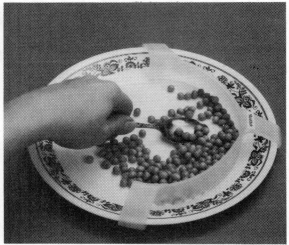

Courtesy of Maddak Inc.

Food bumper.

Food bumpers or **food guards** are snap-on curved rails that fit the side of the plate to keep food from sliding off. They come in two sizes, and are made of polyethylene plastic or stainless steel.

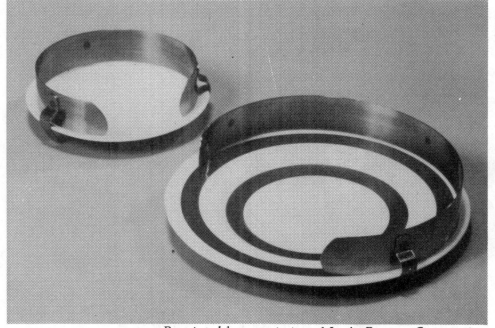

Reprinted by permission of J. A. Preston Corporation.

Food bumpers.

Since the look of a plate can often enhance or detract from a person's appetite, clear food guards, which have been designed to be invisible, help the user get away from that handicapped feeling.

Because it is important to keep the look or the attractiveness of a place setting in mind, a plastic, filmy, non-skid material called dycem is now being used for place mats. However, it is quite expensive. Dycem is available where other aids to independence are sold.

For patients who have lost muscle tone, especially at the sides of their mouth, bibs are in order. A **bib-holder** is a simple gadget to keep the bib snug under the chin. It comes with rust resistant clips with plastic ferrules, and a nylon cord.

Bib hoops are also available commercially, but these can be made just as easily at home. The plastic hoops are threaded through the hem end of a terry cloth, very similar in style to the hoops used to put around the waist to hold an apron.

For those people with severe disabilities, there are many **automatic feeders** on the market. Some are battery-powered and others are operated by chin switches so that quadriplegics can still feed themselves. An electronically acti-vated feeding arm moves the spoon from plate to mouth and back to plate; the height of the arm is adjustable.

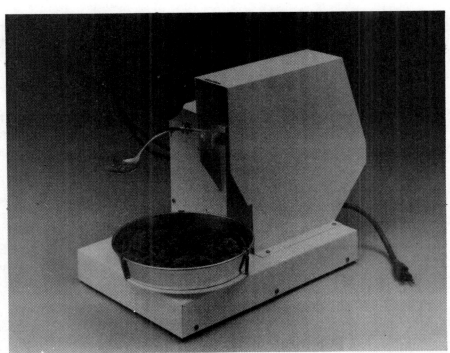

Courtesy of Maddak Inc.

Automatic feeder.

7

BEDROOM AIDS

"In bed we laugh, in bed we cry . . . The near approach, a bed may show, of human bliss to human woe."

Isaac de Benserade

a. BED TYPES

For most people a bed is a place to sleep. But for some, because of a disability, a bed is where they spend a good portion of their waking hours as well.

Beds come in many styles and vary from the very sophisticated, all-electric bed, which costs over $4,000, to the average bed which costs about $300. For the person who is temporarily confined to bed at home, **hospital beds** can be rented from medical supply outlets, the Red Cross, and other service organizations.

For anyone who is confined to bed for a long time, a **waterbed** has some therapeutic value. Unlike the traditional mattress, which supports the body at a few points, the waterbed conforms to the body's shape. The result is that the pressure points are alleviated and bed sores are rarer.

The buoyant support gives a soothing feeling of floating. Sometimes the vinyl-encased, water which can be kept at any temperature, can soothe sore joints.

Early waterbeds waved with every movement, but today's designs control excessive waving. After the first initial surge, the bed settles down. Waterbeds are available in most major centers in Canada and the United States. The cost ranges from $400 to $3,000.

Air beds are fairly new to the marketplace. Designed primarily for burn victims and long-term hospital patients, these beds may prevent infection causing skin loss caused by inability to turn over. However, there are still some bugs to iron out before their design can be accepted on the commercial market as a valuable aid to those suffering disability.

b. ACCESSORIES

If a hospital bed is not available for a patient who requires a lot of care, various alterations can be made to the ordinary bed to make it easier for the person tending the patient. For example, the bed may be raised from the floor so that less bending is required to administer to the patient.

While books are sometimes used to elevate the foot or head of the bed as required, these are not recommended, as they have a tendency to slip. **Risers** are more stable. They come in sets of two or four, in different heights, and cost under $20.

To help the patient sit up in bed, several cushions are often used for support. But they tend to slip and slide with every movement, and need constant attention. **Slant cushions,** which look like a wedge, can remedy this problem. They are available in a variety of washable, print coverings, which help brighten up the room in addition to providing the needed support.

Special **contour pillows** that have been specifically designed to support the neck are also on the market. They can be purchased with liners that are stain and fire resistant but also soft enough for maximum comfort.

A wedge-shape cushion from Switzerland is available to elevate the feet.

An adjustable **foot board** with a spring mechanism for exercising is widely available. It has a foam-cushioned heel support and a velcro strap that makes the device look like a stirrup into which the foot is slipped.

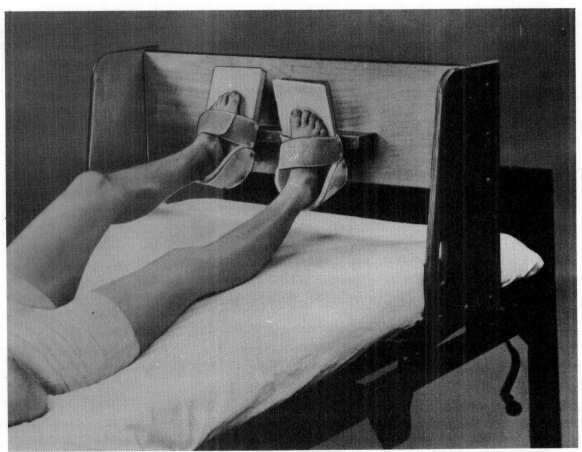

Reprinted by permission of J. A. Preston Corporation, 1985.

Foot board.

The **bed boot** is another aid for those who are confined to bed for long periods. This is a washable plush liner with a velcro strap, and it can be attached to a frame. The bed boot is important in preventing decubiti and equinus deformities.

Not quite as expensive are ordinary **bed socks,** considered a godsend by many elderly. They come in wool or cotton, plain or fancy, and cost less than $10, but a person can knit or crochet a pair for under $2.

The **Roho flotation mattress** is certainly a good bet for long stays in bed. It is filled with air, yet gives the feel of floating on water. However, it is quite expensive — usually more than $2,000.

People confined to bed are sometimes incontinent. For protection, there are specially-made **sheets, pads, and pillowcases** that can be washed at home, or professionally. **Bed soaker pads** can also be purchased individually or by the dozen for increased absorption of moisture.

Transfer boards are very handy for shifting a person from bed to chair. Inexpensive ones can be made at home out of plywood. Attach non-skid strips to the bottom edges.

Bed trays are fairly inexpensive items, especially those made of plastic. These come in various colors and styles. Home-made trays or those made in senior citizen workshops can be geared to the individual's needs.

Dycem is excellent as a place mat or tray cloth. It is a film-like material that can be placed on smooth surfaces to prevent dishes from slipping.

For the at-home patient, over-bed tables, much like those used in institutions, are available. They come with an instant vanity that can be adjusted for height. The vanity is exposed when the top is slipped out of the way.

These over-bed tables have been designed for dining, reading, or writing in bed. They have a tilt top that locks into five different positions. Some have free rolling wheels, while others have a "U" shaped base, permitting it also to be used as an **over-chair table.**

One manufacturer has devised an **able table** — the "everything" table. These able tables can serve as bookholders, easels, lecturns, bed tables and wheelchair trays. They have adjustable aluminum legs and knob settings to adjust the angle and height of the table. Movable elastic straps are an option that can be added for securing items to either the top or the bottom surface of the table. Able tables cost about $50.

Those who have a hearing disability cannot hear an alarm clock and, the flashing light concept is of little use when a person is asleep. So **clocks with vibrating alarms** have been developed to do the job. The remote vibrator is placed under the sleeper's pillow, and is set like any other alarm. At the proper time the pre-set alarm triggers the vibrator which gently shakes the user awake. These special needs clocks are available in various models and cost about $175.

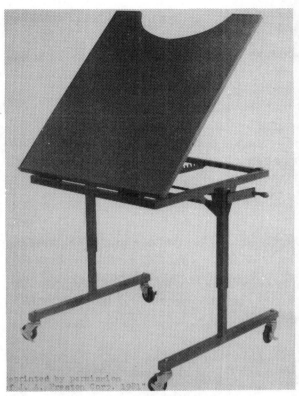

*Reprinted by permission of
J. A. Preston Corporation, 1985.*

Able table.

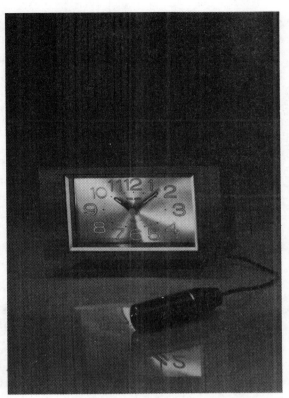

*Reprinted by permission of
J. A. Preston Corporation, 1985.*

Clock with vibrating alarm.

8

BATHROOM AIDS

The bathroom is where we treasure our privacy the most. Unfortunately, it is also where most accidents occur.

Researchers and designers have spent a good deal of time and money adapting bathroom facilities for those who have difficulty because of a handicap. They have designed new articles, revised old ones, and modified others until now we have a wide range of self-helps from toilet seats to arms for those who are unable to cleanse themselves.

a. TOILET AIDS

For many people using a toilet is an impossible task. Researchers have come up with many variations of special toilets from elevated seats that fit over regular toilet seats to more traditional commode models.

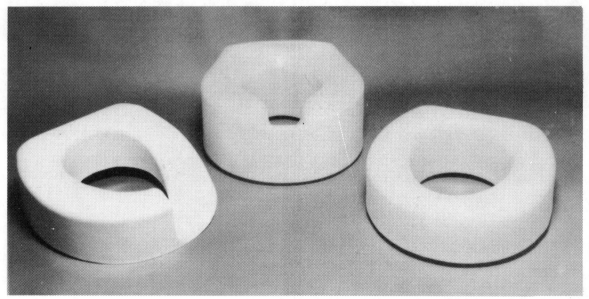

Courtesy of Maddak Inc.

Arthro for hip, elevated, and regular doughnut toilet seats.

The cheapest **raised seat,** made of polypropylene, costs about $30. It is a simple doughnut style which raises the seat level about 4 to 6 inches (10 to 15 cm).

Another model provides a **contoured elevated seat** which gives the user greater hip comfort and security, and places the body in a better position with its front design for proper urine drainage.

52

The **arthro** is a trade name for an elevated seat with either a sloping right or left front side, which permits the user's leg to extend without bending. This seat is elevated 4 to 8 inches (10 to 20 cm), and is also suitable for those who have had a leg amputated.

Because of these elevated seats and the danger of falling from them, toilet safety frames have been designed for the user's protection. They come in many styles, some with just one arm support, others with two; some are attached to the base of the toilet, and some stand free. These frames can be adjusted to various toilet heights, and the support arms, which come singly or in pairs, can be adjusted by push-button controls.

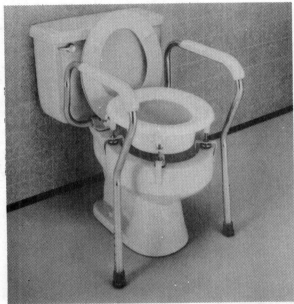

Courtesy of Lumex Inc.   *Courtesy of Maddak Inc.*

Raised toilet with free support frame.

Multi purpose commode-shower-chair hi-level toilet seat and visitor's chair.

There are many models of **toilet raisers.** One in particular looks like an inverted stove-pipe hat with a lower crown. This model can be securely clamped onto regular or elongated bowls, and can be easily removed when other members of the family want to use the facility.

Another design, the **free standing frame** looks much like a walker, except the bars holding the frame together in front are much lower, actually below the toilet bowl level. Non-adjustable frames are a few dollars cheaper than those with adjustable heights, which range in price from $50 up.

Commodes, of course, are portable, and often come with casters on the legs. The most economical ones have an aluminum frame with a white, molded toilet seat and a boilable polyetheylene pail. The plain models sell for about $75.

More elaborate commodes have arms that pivot to allow the user to slide on from the side. These have a brake on the front casters. The commode can be used with a pan, or can be placed over a toilet. It has a back and a lid trap that hides the pail or container when it is not in use. These units cost about $300.

Commodes are manufactured in many other designs: some can be folded up and put away when not needed; others give the impression that they are just an ordinary chair but instead have a lift-off seat cushion. Some commodes have been designed so that they can take on a dual role, for example, they can also be wheeled into the shower and used as a shower chair.

Personal hygiene is another area in which many disabled and elderly experience problems. For one thing, toilet tissue holders are often difficult to reach. To help there is a device that slips onto the commode or support frame; it can be adjusted to any height to suit the user.

Another aid is toilet tongs, made of chrome-plated steel with vinyl-coated ends and handle, the tongs will close around tissue or cotton for cleansing purposes.

Another manufacturer has made a white rubber aid that looks much like a seal with an inverted tail. It snaps onto the toilet seat, and tissue is wrapped around it.

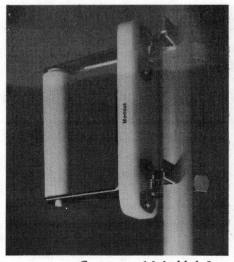

Courtesy of Maddak Inc.

Snap-on toilet tissue holder.

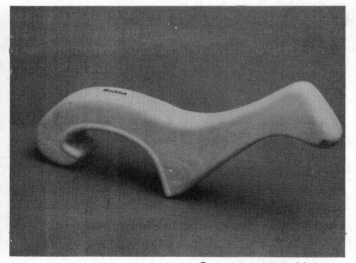

Courtesy of Maddak Inc.

Toilet wipe aid.

b. BATH AND SHOWER AIDS

For those people with extreme disabilities, who cannot manage a bath even with a shower chair, there are **bath lift chairs** which are mounted on a hydraulic hoist.

Actually, the bathroom has a multitude of aids which range from grab bars to sophisticated slings. **Grab bars** or **safety rails** come in different styles and lengths, from a long wall bar, to an angle rail or corner bar.

Security bars are a little different, but serve the same purpose. They clamp onto the open side of the tub. Some will even fit into the old-fashioned gate-legged tubs.

Bathroom safety grips look much like miniature chrome steps as there are three levels of elevation, while the bathtub safety rail is a combination of the "security" rail with a grip frame design much like the front of a walker.

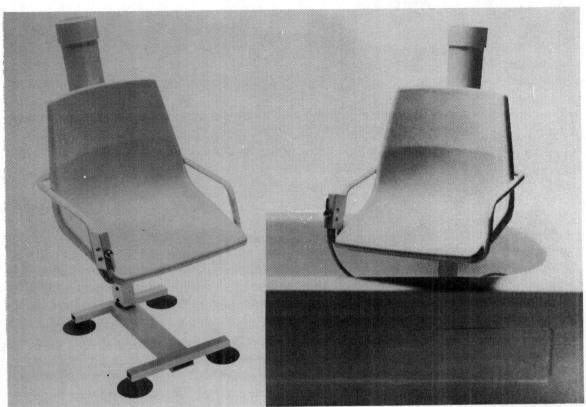

Courtesy of American Stair-Glide Corporation, Grandview, Missouri.

Tubmate™ bath lift.

Bath and shower benches or chairs come in dozens of styles and models, from plain ones which look like camp stools, to those made of aluminum tubing with plastic mesh seats. These range in price from less than $35 to more sophisticated models at $150. Most are equipped with rubber safety feet.

Some designs, like the **padded bench seat** have a transfer tub bench as an auxiliary helper. It sits half outside the tub and half inside, and allows the user the independence of sliding across.

These benches work well with **flexible shower hoses,** which can be purchased at most plumbing and hardware outlets. These hoses will easily reach to the hand level of someone sitting on a bench in the tub. **Special nozzles** operated by a push-button when the user is ready to bathe can make showering a pleasure again for those who have problems with the more traditional ways of showering.

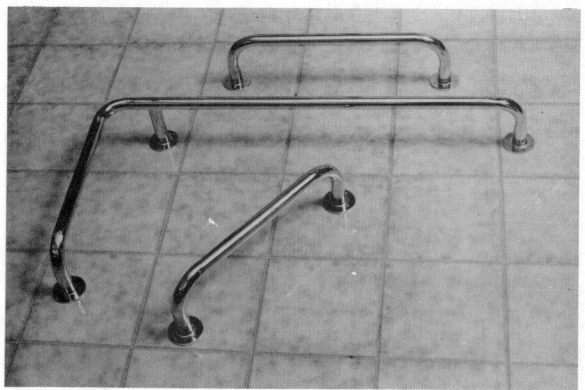

Courtesy of Lumex Inc.

Bathtub safety rails

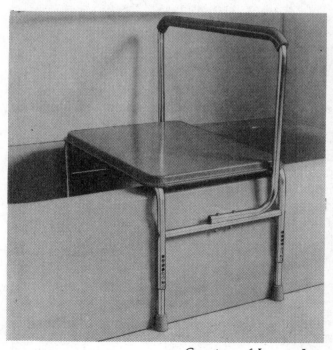

Courtesy of Lumex Inc.
Shower chair.

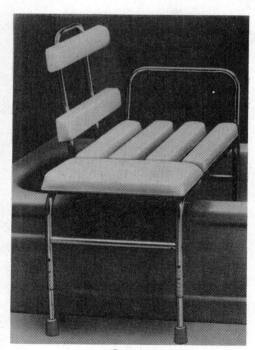

Courtesy of Lumex Inc.
Padded shower seat or bench.

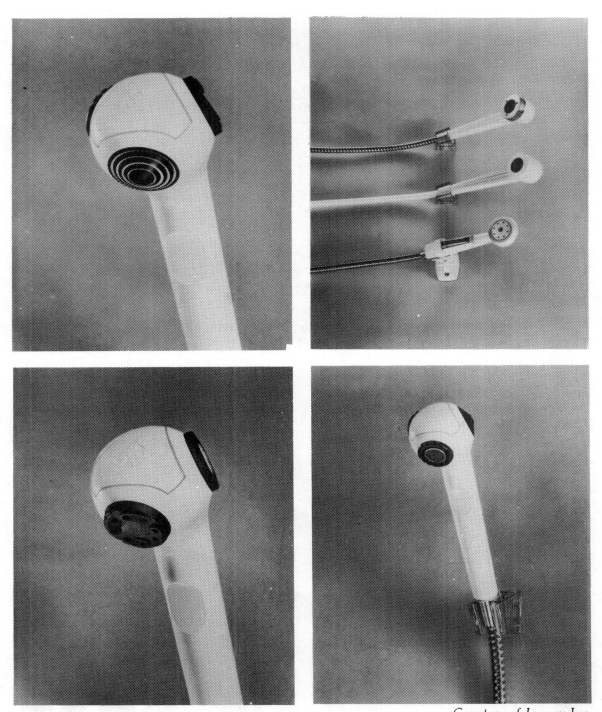

Courtesy of Lumex Inc.

Shower heads.

For bathtub users, the temperature of the water can be a problem. Some older people lose their skin sensitivity and don't realize the heat of the water until they are badly burned. There are several **bath thermometers** on the market;

these change color according to the temperature of the water. This use of color to gauge water temperature is an inexpensive method to monitor the level of heat, especially for a person who has not only lost some of their skin sensitivity, but vision as well.

The color scheme is simple: red means danger, the water is too hot; blue means the water is too cold; and green means it is safe to get in. They are very easy to apply; just remove the adhesive backing and attach to the side of the tub.

Bath stick-ons prevent accidents. They are a non-slip adhesive backed set of decals or strips which can be purchased at hardware and grocery stores. They stick to the bottom of the tub and provide a non-slip tread to make getting in and out of the tub less hazardous. Available in many different colors, these bath stick-ons cost less than $5.

For the person with reaching problems, there are a variety of special bath sponges and brushes. One, the magic soaper, has a sponge attached to the end of a long handle with a pocket to hold the soap.

Another variation of the bath sponge consists of a foot-long aluminum handle with a rubber grip, which has a sponge attached. The angle brush, by means of a wing nut, enables the user to scrub his or her back and legs.

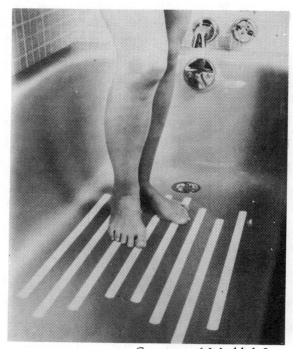

Courtesy of Maddak Inc.

Adhesive safety strips.

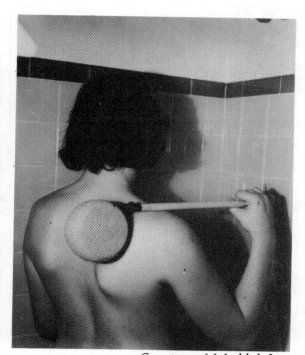

Courtesy of Maddak Inc.

Bath sponge on handle.

The European-style washmitt is easy to make. It is basically a washcloth sewn to form a mitt, into which the user's hand easily slips, eliminating a problem of gripping a brush or bar of soap.

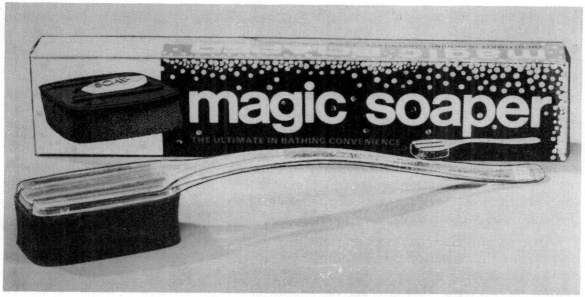

Reprinted by permission of J. A. Preston Corporation.
Magic Soaper.

9

CLOTHING

To look good is to feel good, and people need to feel good about themselves. Since clothing and grooming both play an important part in the way we see ourselves, naturally they affect our well-being.

Just because people have problems does not mean they have to look frumpy or untidy. Attractive, comfortable, and reasonably priced geriatric clothing has been designed especially for seniors and the disabled. There are outlets in most major cities in North America with mail order services to back them up.

Supplying clothing for the elderly and those with special needs has long been recognized as a commendable, but not necessarily profitable business. But with the senior population increasing by leaps and bounds, geriatric and special needs clothing is becoming a rapidly expanding and lucrative industry.

In Ontario, Canada, geriatric clothing outlets are taking to the road; mobile units travel to nursing homes and homes for the aged, taking their products to those who lack the mobility to get out and shop. Primarily, these clothing outlets specialize in fashionable, attractive, adaptable clothing that will stand up to the rigors of industrial washing.

Before this type of marketing, the only outlets for special needs clothing were mail order houses like Wings of Vocational Guidance and Rehabilitation Services of Cleveland, Ohio and Fashion Able of Rocky Hill, New Jersey.

Wings, one of the oldest and largest innovative rehabilitation agencies in the world, was the pioneer in this field of clothing and aids for the disabled. A member of the United Way and the Federation of Community Planning, it has been manufacturing special clothing since 1962. For $2. they will send a catalogue showing designs that are manufactured and stocked for immediate delivery to customers. The order forms, which accompany the catalogue, feature charts to indicate exactly how to measure for made-to-measure garments when a special design is necessary. These measurements must be accurate, as there are no refunds or exchanges on purchases, and all orders must be prepaid.

Wings features contemporary styles in small, medium, large, and extra large, at reasonable prices. In their list of accomplishments, they note that they have "designed a sports jacket for a paraplegic, created a fashionable wardrobe for a very modern young women with leg braces on crutches, and designed slacks with a different right and left leg for a stroke victim."

Most of Wing's standard line is also available through Sears, Roebuck and Co.'s General Catalogue.

Fashion Able of Rocky Hill, New Jersey, was conceived by Mrs. VanDavid Odell. Her concern stemmed from the problems experienced by people who were unable to purchase undergarments to suit their needs. She decided to design and produce her own line for those with physical handicaps and other limitations.

The growth of Mrs. Odell's venture has made Fashion Able a recognized name across North America. And now, instead of just clothing, hundreds of other products have been added to the company's mail order shopping service.

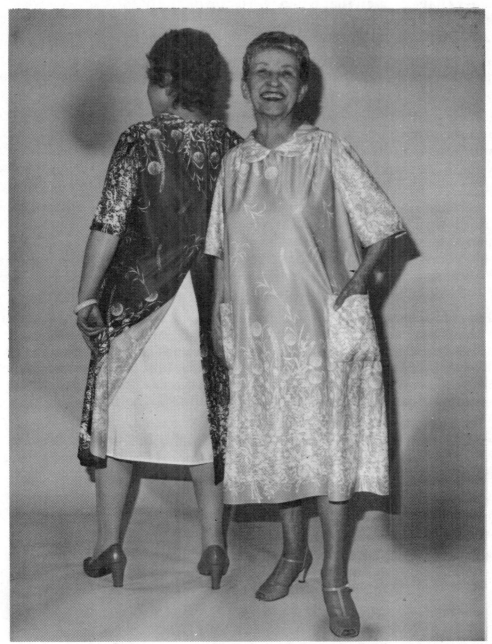

Courtesy of Comfort Clothing, Kingston Inc.

Easy to wear back-opening dress.

Her early catalogue featured brassieres with covered velcro strips instead of more traditional hooks and eyes; slips with long zipper fronts that women could step into; and girdles with zippered front panels.

Many of Fashion Able's items are almost impossible to find elsewhere: sanitary skirt shields; knee warmers; wraparound garter belts; and isotoner driving gloves. These gloves were developed at the Einstein Medical Center, and researchers have proven that when worn during the night, they relieve morning stiffness and swelling in the hands. These gloves come in one size, which fits all. They are washable and cost about $12.

Women's union suits are also featured in Fashion Able's catalogues. These are one-piece knits with complete coverage to the knee, built-up straps, and an open seat. They come in various sizes and cost about $10.

At Kingston, Ontario, based on the findings of a community college study of the special clothing needs of senior citizens, Lorraine Heaney and Elinor Rush formed a non-profit organization called Comfort Clothing Service. In less than five years the company found a market across Canada, and in 1983 they formed an employee-owned corporation called Comfort Clothing Kingston Inc.

There are certain guidelines that must be adhered to when developing geriatric clothing. The needs of the wearer are of paramount importance. The emphasis should be on function and comfort as well as fashion. Clothing should always move with the body, so the cut of the garment is very important. A crotch that is too short, a sleeve that binds, or a collar that is too tight only compounds a problem.

Many older people prefer the older styles, which feature garments that flow rather than restrict. In choosing any style, it is important to remember that pleats in the back of a skirt, pleats in the center back of a blouse, or pleats in the side of a jacket, give added room. A tuck of any kind provides extra cloth for greater freedom of movement. For instance, raglan or kimono sleeves allow more shoulder freedom than regular, set-in ones. Gathered neck-lines also help play down features such as a sagging bustline or a dowager's hump.

People with special needs should avoid dangling belts or ties, hard to fasten buttons or loops, skirt or pant lengths that can cause falls, or loopy accessories that can catch on protruding surfaces.

By emphasizing positive features and making allowances for problem areas, designers have come up with a highly adaptable line of clothing that not only perks up the spirits of the wearer, but lends itself to independence.

No product has made a greater impact on clothing designed for special needs than velcro. Made of nylon, one side of a velcro fastener consists of tiny hook-like fibers, hardly discernible to the naked eye, while the other surface consists of minute loops. When the two are pressed together, they lock; when peeled apart, they unlock.

Since velcro is a man-made fabric, care must be taken not to expose it to high temperatures when washing or ironing. Velcro can be purchased for a few cents at most sewing departments, and comes in black, white, and beige.

Magnetic fasteners have also received wide acceptance, as they require little muscle tone to fasten or pull apart.

Buttons have not been forgotten in geriatric wear. They tend to be larger than most buttons, with a wide rim, making them easier to grasp. For those who have trouble with buttons of any kind, there are **button loops** and **button hooks.** Usually these items come with a small built-up handle, and a tapered, wire-thread loop which goes through the button hole to loop over the button and pull it back through the opening. These cost about $8 to $10.

Zippers, long a frustration for those with grip or grasp problems, have generally been replaced by velcro. For a while it was thought that separating zippers might be a replacement for difficult shirt buttons, but people with special needs have trouble getting them started.

However, on clothing where zippers do exist, **zipper pulls** are invaluable. There are several on the market. A long-reach zipper pull eliminates the problem of hard-to-reach closures. The "pull" is a metal hook, which goes through the zipper tab. This hook is attached to a plastic cord with a ring at the end. The user pulls up on the ring to close the zipper, pulls down to open. This can also be made at home by using cord, a heavy-duty paper clip, and a metal ring.

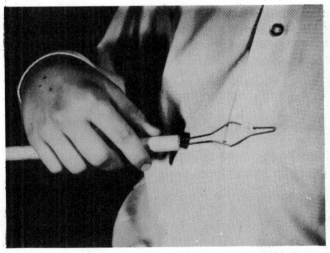

Courtesy of Maddak Inc.

Button loop.

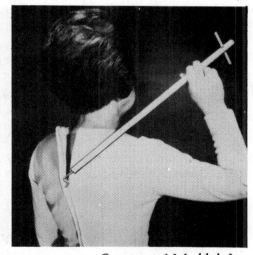

Courtesy of Maddak Inc.

Zipper pull.

There are also **short zipper pulls** designed for people who have difficulty grasping pull tabs. These come in two sizes, one with a regular handle and one with a built-up handle.

Ring zipper pulls, which remain permanently attached to the zipper tab, usually come in packages of three. A user just clips it through the hole in the zipper tab, and the large ring makes zipping up or down a little easier.

Men certainly have not been forgotten in the geriatric line: **pants, shirts, and socks** have been manufactured in adaptive styles. For those who must wear leg-braces, zippers can be sewn into the side seam of pant legs. The pants can also be interlined to guard against the extra wear of the brace. Velcro closings are an excellent substitute for fly zippers for men who have the added problem of grasp or limited muscle power in hands or wrists.

CLOTHING

In their catalogue, Wings shows an adaptive line of men's **slacks** which have a drop front, drop back, or both. They feature an interband that keeps slacks in place while the front or back is lowered, but which still allows freedom of function the rest of the time. These slacks have false flies, velcro-fastened waistbands, and optional seam openings for people with braces.

Shirts, too, have received their share of attention. They feature set-in sleeves, extra room in the armholes, and velcro cuffs and front openings. Shirts made with this extra roominess are also available with the traditional snap or button closures.

Many suppliers of geriatric clothing feature old-fashioned **nightshirts** for men. These garments are made of comfortable flannelette and other woven fabrics, and cost about the same as a regular pair of pajamas. Some styles have twin pockets, easy-on sleeves, and a shirt-tail hemline.

Adaptive line pajamas have an added feature that regular styles do not: they come with one, two, or even three sets of bottoms for each top.

For men in wheelchairs who want to look stylish, Leinenweber Inc., custom tailors, have done a great deal to provide comfortable and attractive clothing. They have developed a system of tailoring suits and coats specifically for men who must sit, by eliminating material where it is not needed, and adding it where it is, with the overall objective being to achieve comfort.

Jobst-Stride is the trademark of a line of **support socks** and **stockings** designed to apply pressure to the legs. This relieves fatigue and discomfort common to the legs of people who stand a lot. They have a puffy, loop-toe closure which assures the wearer of a no-ridge, flat seam.

Several manufacturers feature lines of socks and stockings which, while not specifically designed for people with problems, do adapt better to certain needs. There are also the regular **panty hose, knee-highs,** and special **stay-ups.** These stay-ups can be worn without garters, are free of wrinkles, and have no elastic from top to toe, although the toe is reinforced for longer wear. All of these styles come in small, medium, and large.

Incontinence is a big worry for many older people. For one thing, it prohibits travel — even going to the store can be a hazardous experience. Consequently, many innovations in this field now provide protection and security. Pants for the incontinent come in styles for both men and women.

Kanga pants feature a pouch or crotch pocket at the front where absorbent pads can be inserted. They have washable liners which can be purchased in quantities of 20 for about $10 and in lots of 200 for $75. These kanga liners can be inserted or removed without removing the pants.

There are also **maxi-plus pants** which are made of elastic thread. Since the stitching is quite loose, these pants are airy and pliable. They have two ribbons woven into the front to hold the liners firmly in place.

A maxi-pocket pad looks like a bag, and has been designed to slip over the penis to collect small, accidental leakages of urine. They are available by the carton, 25 for $20.

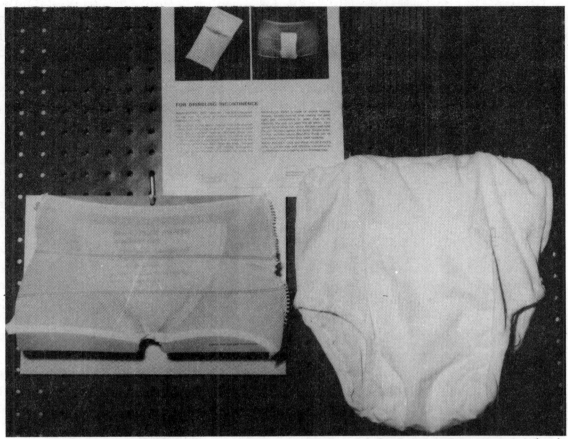

Courtesy of Doncaster Medical.

Maxi-Plus pants (left) and Kanga pants.

For women, there are several styles of **protective pants** from those not much bigger than bikinis to larger bloomer styles which have elastic at the legs and around the top. These pants are made of rayon, lined with plastic, and come in fitted and dome styles. The dome style allows the pants to lie flat like a diaper, making them easy to put on or take off.

There is the additional problem of patients who unintentionally expose themselves. The Posey Company of Arcadia, California, has come up with **locking pants** which have shoulder straps and a hidden buckle to keep the pants in place. When unlocked, the pants are easily removed. These garments can be worn as ordinary clothing, or over the user's own clothing. They are available in long and short styles for both men and women.

Modesty aprons also protect against accidental exposure. One style is like a lap rug, which covers the person when sitting; another is like an apron with a full skirt, which can wrap around the person's waist. It can be a colorful garment with the added utility of a pocket, and need not reflect the use for which it was designed.

Modesty aprons are fastened with velcro tabs, or tied at the waist. Good for use indoors and out, their cost is a small price to pay for dignity.

10

GROOMING AND DRESSING AIDS

German poet Johann Christoph von Schiller said, "Everyone stamps his own value on himself." And this axiom is never more true than in the lives of people faced with problems in grooming and dressing. In their own eyes, their value is stamped on their own efforts to help themselves.

Often, it is the little things that bring about the greatest frustrations; these little things accumulate until they become destructive to the person. Dressing oneself can be a regular obstacle course if a person cannot bend, reach, or grasp. Therefore, items that help in grooming and dressing rate highly on the list of aids for independence.

Just combing your hair can be a chore if you can't raise your arms. **Combs and brushes** with built-up handles, combs with extra long handles, or handles that curve are enough for some handicapped people, but others need more sophisticated aids. One such aid is a comb attached to a long plastic arm that bends at two points: a wrist and an elbow. Some models are battery-powered.

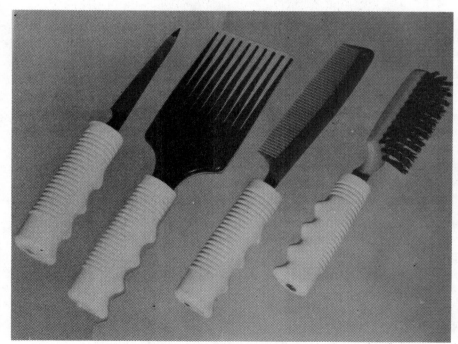

Courtesy of Maddak Inc.

Built-up handles on grooming aids.

However, a homemade unit, which is a comb with a handle pushed onto a styrofoam ball, can provide better grasp. If the foam is not available, then the handle can simply be wrapped with gauze and bound with adhesive tape.

A hair brush can be adapted to suit the user's needs. Insert it into a bicycle handlebar grip and fill the grip with wet plaster. When the plaster sets, a good, built-up handle has been made at a fraction of the cost of a commercial product.

Regular, **closed-cell foam** can be purchased in cylinder rolls for fashioning built-up handles for aids at home. This foam looks much like solidified shaving foam in a cylinder mold with a hole running through the center. When cut into the desired length, the foam can be rammed, jammed or worked over ordinary utensil handles, allowing the user a larger surface to grip.

For people who cannot grip a handle of any kind, **straps with velcro** closings can be attached to the back of a brush, providing good maneuverability. Also on the market is a **finger ring hairbrush** made of soft plastic. It is octagonal rather than the traditional rectangular shape. The user simply slides a finger through the ring of the brush. It also makes a good shampoo brush.

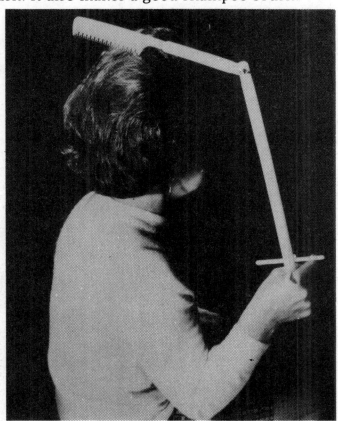

Courtesy of Maddak Inc.
Comb on handle.

A **quad brush** is similar in design. It is wider than the normal brush, and has a "slip-hand-in" holder.

For women who like to do their own hair, but who have only limited use of their arms (like a stroke victim), special **hair rollers** have been designed. These have tiny, nylon hooks that catch and hold the hair on the roller without the help of clips or pins.

Shampoo basins, which are inflatable rings that fit around the neck of the user and provide a soft surface to rest the neck on, make washing and rinsing easier. A hand-held hose sprays water over the hair, and the used water drains from the tray through a tube into a basin or pail on the floor.

Cleaning teeth can also be a chore, so **toothbrushes** have also been adapted to suit special needs. While those with built-up and extended handles are available on the commercial market, toothbrushes, like combs and hair brushes, can also be adapted at home at nominal cost. For example, a wide elastic band can be taped to a toothbrush handle for people who cannot grasp a small item.

For cleaning dentures, a toothbrush can be placed into a base with suction cups to secure it to the counter top; the user simply rubs the dentures against the brush. A much cheaper version that accomplishes the same purpose can be made by securing a nail brush to the counter with a suction cup.

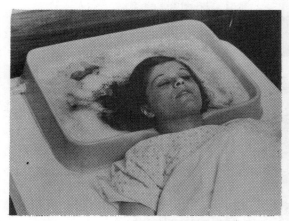

Courtesy of Maddak Inc.

Shampoo basin.

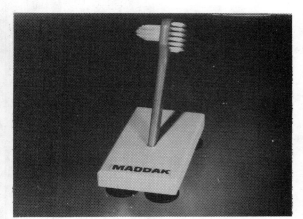

Courtesy of Maddak Inc.

Dental brush in suction holder.

Getting the most out of a tube of toothpaste even with two hands is not easy. For those with limited muscle tone, a great deal of paste can go to waste because it cannot be squeezed or rolled up the tube. **Toothpaste tube squeezers** have been made commercially, but home varieties will work just as well. A dowel fitted with a handle provides the key-like unit around which the toothpaste tube can be rolled.

Even using a **spray deodorant** can be a chore. A device that looks much like an inverted L-bar can be anchored to the side of the spray can, and held in place with a clamp. The inverted base of the "L" lies over the spray valve, and when pressed against the valve, the spray is released. Pressure can be applied to the bar with the flat of the hand, or the fingers.

While the **electric razor** has made shaving a lot easier, some people are unable to hold one. Manufacturers have designed a vinyl-coated, steel handle which can be bent to fit the user's hand. A foam pad inside the handle helps to grip the shaver and minimize vibrations.

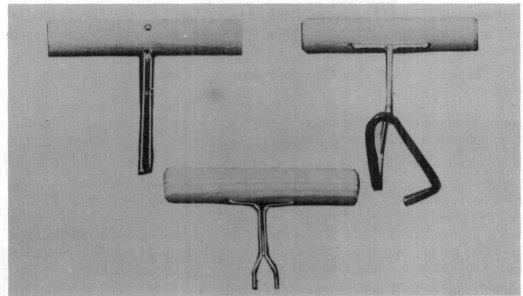

Courtesy of Maddak Inc.

Toothpaste tube squeezers.

An automobile seat belt buckle and webbing can secure a shaver to the user's hand.

Goose neck mirrors can be maneuvered to different heights and angles to suit the need. Similarly, mirrors on swivel arms are of great assistance.

Even cutting nails can be a trial for those with muscle tone, reaching or grasp limitations. Ordinary **nail clippers** can be fixed with a dowel handle that has a slit in the end. The nail clippers can then be anchored in this slit with a small screw.

On the commercial market is another type of nail clipper, which looks much like a paper stapler. It is anchored to a base and the base in turn is anchored to a surface by suction cups on the underside.

An ordinary nail file can also be secured by suction cups to any flat surface. The file is inverted through loops of certain styles of cups. Equally useful is a small piece of wood with a slit in the end, into which a nail file is inserted and secured.

Blowing the nose can be a big problem. People who cannot reach up to their noses must use tongs or reachers to hold their handkerchiefs. But to blow the nose in this way requires a great deal of skill — not just in opening the tongs, but in opening them just wide enough to cover the nose and not so wide as to drop the handkerchief. It is an art in itself.

Adaptive clothing has certainly helped people dress themselves, but sometimes even specially designed clothing is not the whole answer.

Dressing sticks are made of metal or wood (wood is cheaper) and come in various lengths. Some have only a single wire hook on one end, usually with a rubber tip on the other end. All dressing sticks allow the user to reach over a shoulder with one arm, hook a garment, lift it and swing it across the back, and insert the other arm into a sleeve. The rubber tip on the other end of the dressing stick has a rough, burr surface which enables the user to grasp sheer materials like silks and satins.

Dressing sticks are available at medical supply outlets, and range in price from $8 to $15.

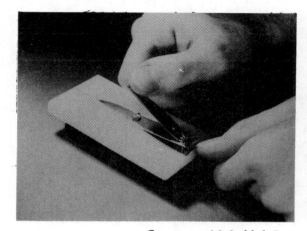

Courtesy of Maddak Inc.

Firmly anchored nail clipper.

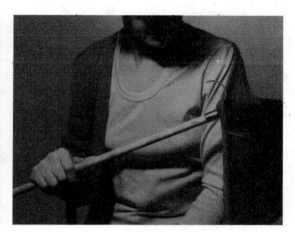

Courtesy of Maddak Inc.

Dressing stick.

Reachers are another big help in dressing. With their magnetic or pincer-like mouths, they can assist the user in clipping on ties or picking up items from the floor. However, long wooden tongs perform the same function and are much less expensive.

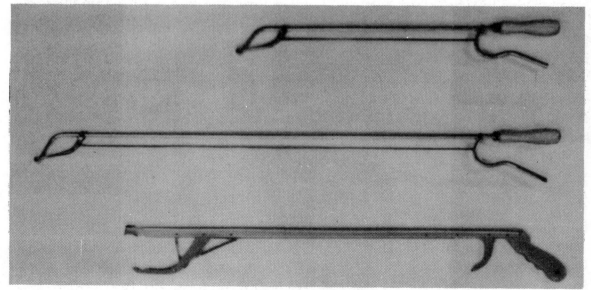

Reprinted by permission of J. A. Preston Corporation.

Reachers.

Panty or skirt aids are simply two wide bands of elastic or webbed material attached to hand loops or sticks. The bands are clipped to the garment, which is then dropped to the floor; the garment can easily be stepped into and pulled up with minimal bending required. The belt-like attachment is simply released when the garment is on.

Stocking aids come in many sizes and styles. Some are designed only for panty hose, while others are designed for multiple uses. Most are made from a soft plastic like that used in detergent bottles, only softer.

One aid, made of butyrate flexible plastic is made especially for support hose. Butyrate plastic has a stronger base and, although malleable, it still holds its shape under the squeezing pressure of support hose.

Most of these aids have garters that are fastened to the top of the hose, which is stretched over a plastic calf or foot-shaped form. This form, attached to a long arm, can be held on the floor, allowing the user to place her feet inside and pull the hose up. The garters are then released and the form removed.

For people who have had hip surgery, **sock aids** are available. Socks are attached to garter clips and pulled up. The garters are released by a simple downward push on the long arm attachment, which looks something like two long chopsticks. Circular hand guards provide a grip along the smooth arm surface; the plastic covered hook on the other end is designed to push or pull.

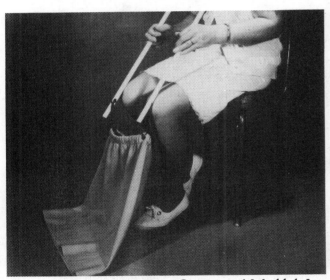

Courtesy of Maddak Inc.

Panty, skirt or slip aid.

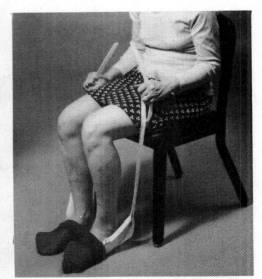

Courtesy of Maddak Inc.

Panty hose aid.

It is possible to fashion a homemade sock aid from heavy-duty plastic containers to which clothes pins and webbing are attached for pulling socks into place. While these are not usually strong enough for support hose, these homemade devices do work on lighter stockings and socks.

For putting on pants without bending, there is an aid made of curved plastic or metal which has garters attached to the pants. Long tabs allow the user to pull up the pants from the floor.

For people who are unable to bend, putting on shoes and boots can be difficult. Extra long **shoe horns,** 24 inches to 36 inches (61 to 91 cm) in length, will aid the user in managing this normally easy task. Plastic units are inexpensive, about $4 to $5, while chrome-plated ones in extra long lengths cost in the neighborhood of $35.

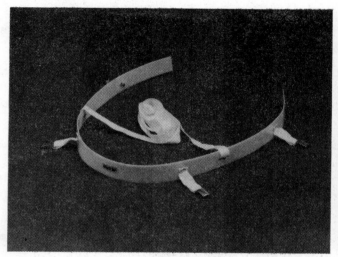

Courtesy of Maddak Inc.
Trouser aid.

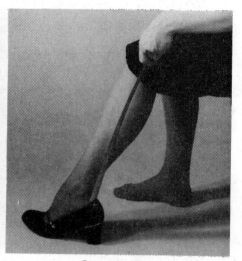

Courtesy of Maddak Inc.
Long shoe horn.

Boot jacks, a throwback from pioneer days, have been redesigned for those people who cannot bend, or who cannot grasp strongly enough to remove shoes or boots. They are often made of wood (there are many variations), and are rectangular in shape. Boot jacks are elevated at one end, with a "U" cut into that end where the boot heel is inserted. By pulling up on the heel, the boot or shoe will slip off.

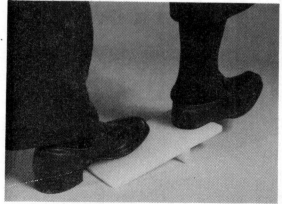

Courtesy of Maddak Inc.
Boot jack.

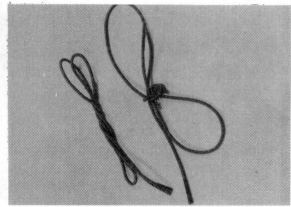

Courtesy of Maddak Inc.
Elastic shoe laces.

Shoe laces, which are quite a problem for those who lack mobility in their fingers, can be managed in two ways. One is to use elastic laces, which permit laced shoes to be slipped on or off without untying them. The second solution is to use **no-bows.** By pinching the ends of the fastener while pulling on the knob, laces are tightened; to loosen laces, the ends of the fastener are pinched.

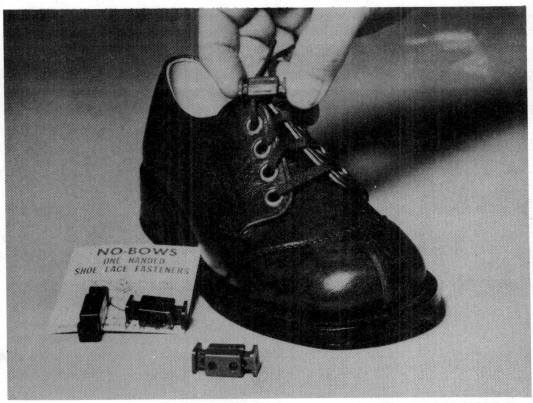

Courtesy of Maddak Inc.

No-bow shoe laces.

11

EXERCISE

Gerontologists tell us that the nearest thing we have to the fountain of youth is exercise. Exercise not only promotes physical health, but helps us work off frustrations and stress, and gives us a feeling of psychological well-being.

Yet those with disabilities find that exercise, in the traditional sense, is not always possible. Jogging, walking or cycling are beyond their physical capabilities. Therefore different forms of exercise must be devised. Afflicted muscles and joints must be kept limber, and the circulatory system must be stimulated.

Exercise apparatus come in all styles, shapes, and sizes from a simple rubber ball to sophisticated bicycle exercisers and treadmills.

Several aids have been developed for stroke victims and arthritis sufferers, but none has taken the place of the **rubber ball** for exercising fingers, hands, and wrists. Manufacturers have taken the ball a step further. It has now been shaped to fit the hand, and sometimes comes with a wrist-attached strap, so that if the ball drops, it will not roll away. This, like many other aids, can be made from materials at home for a fraction of the retail cost.

Playing the piano or organ is also good exercise for arthritic fingers, and quilting and needlepoint are no longer restricted to women.

While **palm grips** and **cones** are helpful to those people who dig their fingernails into their palms after being hit with a stroke, they can also be used as a gentle hand exercise. They can be held in place by an adjustable strap that fits across the back of the hand.

These cones or grips are usually stuffed with kodel and covered with absorbent terry cloth, which can be slipped off for washing.

There is also a **finger contrature cushion,** which is actually a narrow rectangular block of foam about the width of a hand. It has four concaves scooped out of its upper edge. Placed in the hand this contrature cushion allows the concaves to comfortably separate the fingers as they bend forward.

Exercise putty is a flexible exercise material that is used in the treatment of finger and hand problems. Manipulating the putty between the fingers is an effective flexing exercise for the hand muscles.

Hand Gym is the trade name of a product supplied by Maddak Inc. It is a triangular-shaped device made of plastic, with plates, rods, and rubber bands. It is designed specifically to arrest hand deformities and to keep pain to a minimum during use. This device was clinically tested at the Institute of Rehabilitation Medicine of the New York University Medical Center. It can be adjusted to all hand sizes. Many of the parts, including the rods, cushions, and bands, are replaceable.

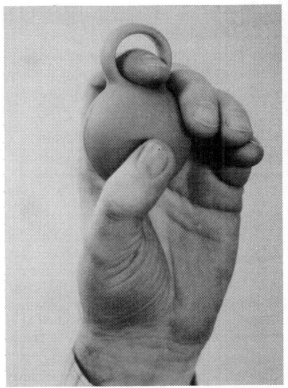

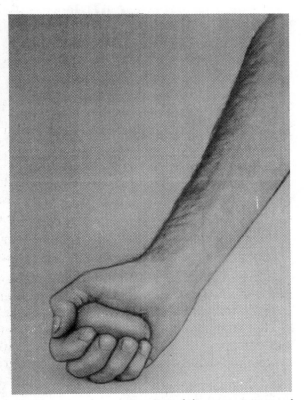

*Reprinted by permission of
J. A. Preston Corporation.*

Palm grip.

*Reprinted by permission of
J. A. Preston Corporation.*

Exercise putty.

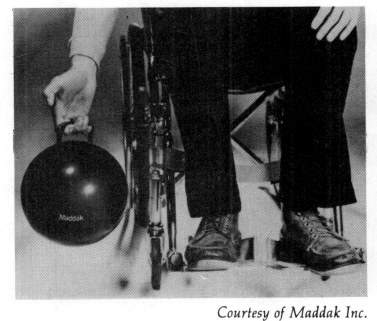

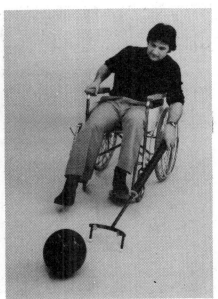

Courtesy of Maddak Inc.

Bowling ball with hand grip.

Courtesy of Maddak Inc.

Bowling ball pusher.

Bowling is an exercise that can be enjoyed by all ages despite finger-grip problems. A **handle grip** allows the bowler to firmly grasp the ball; this grasp handle retracts completely when the ball is set in motion.

Another device used in bowling is the **bowling ball pusher.** Instead of throwing the ball down the alley, it is pushed with this device, somewhat as in shuffleboard. The device looks like a fork with a center tine missing. The ball pusher is supplied with a built-up extension handle to allow its use from a standing or sitting position.

Bowling ramps have been designed for those with very limited use of hands and arms. A bowling partner or assistant lifts the ball onto the frame, and the bowler sets it in motion. These frames may be used by either a sitting or standing bowler.

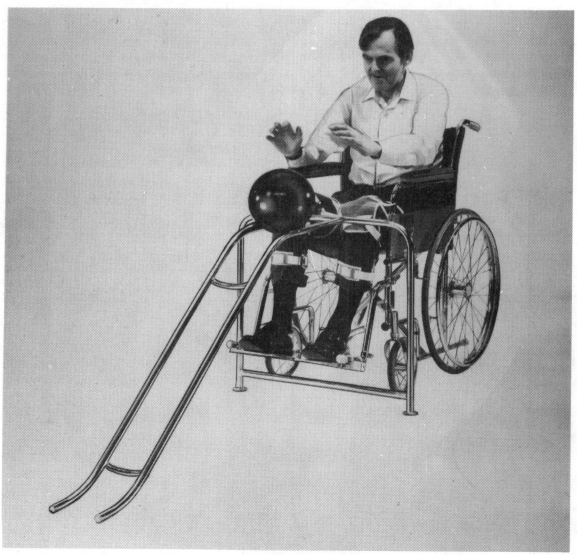

Reprinted by permission of J. A. Preston Corporation.

Bowling ramp.

12

LEISURE

While spare minutes are the gold dust of time, too many spare minutes can drag into hours, days, and weeks. They can shatter the morale of a person whose life is plagued with nothing but spare minutes. There are numerous aids available that can help seniors or disabled persons enjoy their leisure time.

Although not recommended by health professionals smoking is still a favorite way for many people to relax. However, just holding a cigarette or pipe can be a problem for those who cannot maintain a grip. To offset their handicap, **smoking robots** have been developed to assist the smoker. These robots consist of a long plastic tube attached to a sectioned cigarette holder. One part of the holder is attached to the end of the tube, which can be clamped to the frame of a chair so the user can take a puff with just a turn of the head. As the cigarette burns down, the ashes fall into an attached ash tray. When the butt is finished, it is released by a spring action ejector.

Medical supply stores, and some variety and specialty stores, carry **ash trays** with suction cup bases. These are minimal in cost, and preferable to breakable glass or ceramic models. These range in price from $3 to $13.

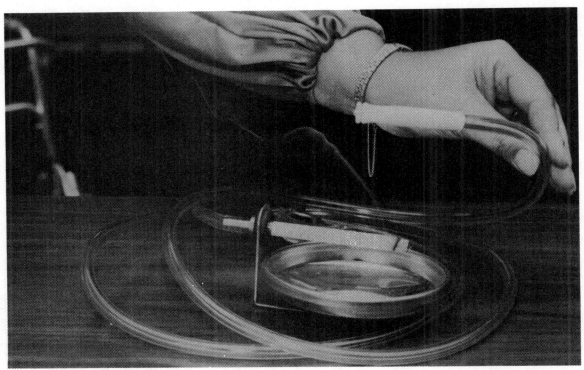

Courtesy of Doncaster Medical and London Free Press, Morris Lamont.
Smoking robot.

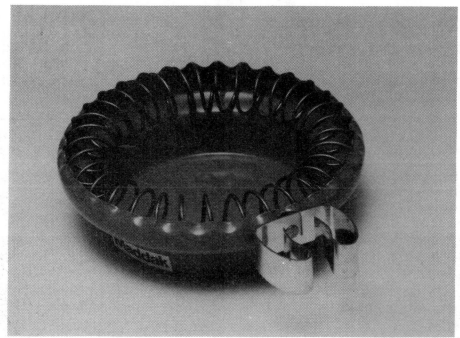

Courtesy of Maddak Inc.

Safety clip-on ash tray.

Even though they can hold a cigarette, many older people will accidentally drop live ashes, which can start a fire. To prevent clothes from catching fire, to protect furniture, and even to prevent ashes from rolling onto the rug, **fire retardant aprons** have been developed by Nor-Stan Institutional Products of Scarborough, Ontario. Several other companies produce similar garments with various adaptations.

Nor-Stan's aprons are 100% fiberglass, and classified as non-combustible by underwriters' laboratories. They are machine washable and dryable, and will not stretch or shrink.

For easier use, they have velcro neck closures, and are equipped with waist straps so they will stay in place. The average cost is less than $10.

a. READING AND WRITING AIDS

Many older people are avid readers, and while they now have the time, they may not have the money to spend on books or magazines. Libraries, of course, are an excellent source of reading materials. Many libraries have a volunteer delivery service for shut-ins, or for those who cannot manage to climb the steps at most library entrances.

Besides the regular lines of books, most libraries stock large print books. They are available in many subject areas, but because of the high cost of producing them, inventories are limited. It is easy to check on what is available. If specific materials are not on hand, the library will often order them through regional library systems.

The pleasure of reading, though, is often denied people because of their physical problems. For those who have difficulty turning pages, there are **hand-held page turners.** And for those who cannot grasp a book, various types of **bookholders** have been designed. They range from simple designs, which cost only a few dollars, to more sophisticated designs with automatic page turners, which cost several hundred dollars.

The more sophisticated holders come with battery-operated page turners that will turn a page simply by touch; in fact, some are so sensitive that they can be activated by the tongue. These are available from medical outlet stores.

For bedridden patients who want to read or watch television, **bedspecs** provide just the right angle of vision. Approved by ophthalmologists, bedspecs are readily adjustable to head width, and can be worn over regular glasses.

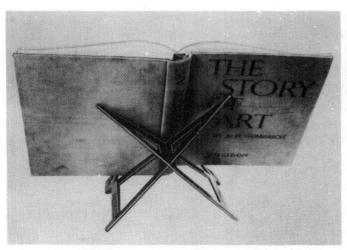

Courtesy of Maddak Inc.

Page turner.

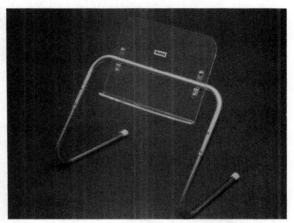

Courtesy of Maddak Inc.

Tubular bookholder.

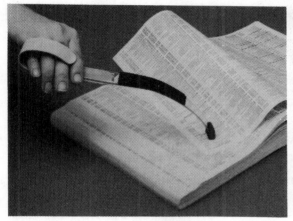

Courtesy of Maddak Inc.

Bookholder.

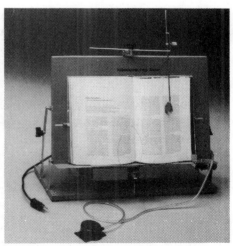

Courtesy of Maddak Inc.

Automatic page turner.

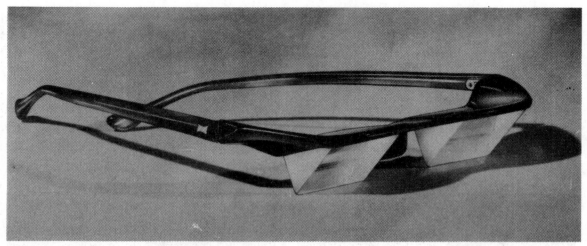

Courtesy of Maddak Inc.

Bedspecs.

For some people, **talking books** (tape cassettes) provide a satisfying alternative to reading. While relatively new on the North American market, talking books have been sold in Great Britain for some time under the giant EMI recording group. The concept is not new, as institutes for the blind have been producing them for years, but mass marketing to the general public is new.

Thanks to this electronic innovation, people can listen to stars of stage and screen read the classics or current authors read their own works. John Gielgud reading *Hamlet* and John LeCarre reading *Tinker, Tailor, Soldier, Spy* show the range of talking books. These "book" cassettes can be played on most cassette players, and cost under $15.

Writing letters is a form of leisure for many people, but if a person cannot hold a pen, or keep the paper from slipping, the enjoyment is lost. For those limited to the use of one hand, a **magnetic holder** holds the paper so it won't slip. This writing pad straps on, and has a magnetic holding force of about 15 pounds (6.8 kg) and can be increased by the addition of paper, or decreased by the removal of paper.

For some people, an ordinary clipboard from any stationery department will be enough to hold paper in place, especially if the problem is the limitation of using one hand, rather than a problem with grasp.

There are many devices for holding a pencil if grasp is the problem. These range from a velcro band with a palm pocket to holders similar to those used for holding a spoon or knife to build-up materials like **Gripkit** from England. Gripkit works on the same premise as plaster of paris. It comes in two-part plastic pouches which, when mixed together, will mold to any shape and stick to almost anything. It is available through medical supply outlets.

Again, to aid in writing, there is a ball with a hole through it. A pen is placed through the hole and clamped in place. This provides a gripping area for the user.

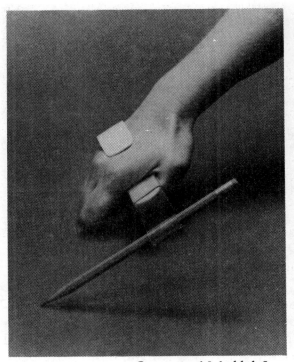

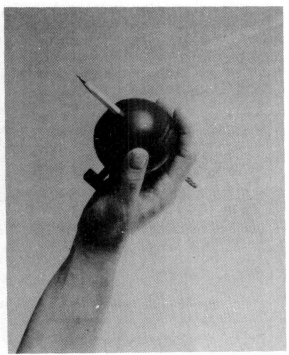

Courtesy of Maddak Inc.

Pencil holder.

Courtesy of Maddak Inc.

Pencil in ball for easy grip.

b. GAMES

There are many board games to pass leisure hours, including dominoes and crokinole. They have been redesigned in new sizes and shapes to accommodate player's disabilities.

Checker games with pegs instead of flat-sided checkers are excellent for relaxation, and they help improve eye and hand co-ordination. To "king" a checker man, the peg is simply inverted as the opposite end is painted a different color.

Tic-tac-toe has been adapted for those with special needs. This game comes with a large board and self-stick labels marked X and O.

Card games are still one of the best ways of passing time. For people who cannot see or hold regular playing cards, there are decks of cards with enlarged faces and numbers, or decks with cards double or triple the size of normal playing ones. For the person living alone, solitaire is still a good bet, and there are books available that describe dozens of ways to play the game.

For people with grip problems, there are various **cardholders** on the market. They range from the simple wooden frame with a grooved lip to those made of two metal disks between which the cards are held. A few models have a flexible steel clamp that secures the unit to a table edge.

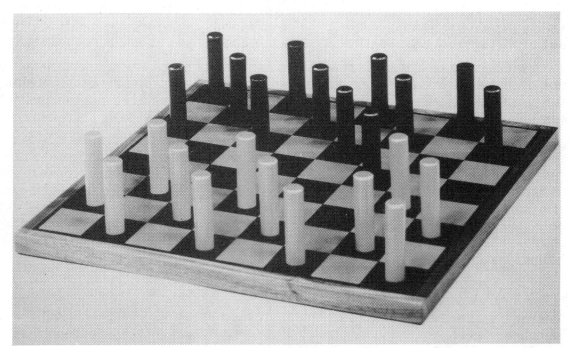

Reprinted by permission of J. A. Preston Corporation.

Checker game with pegs.

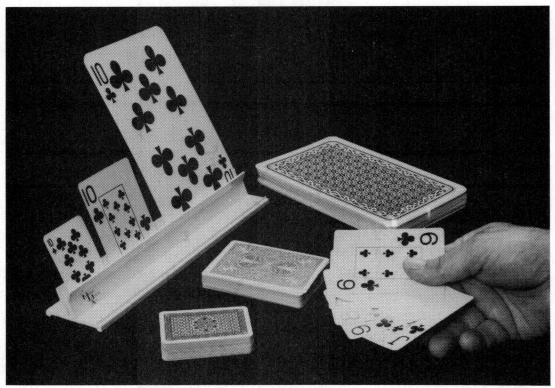

Courtesy of Maddak Inc.

Playing card holders.

Card shufflers are also available, and they are ideal for those with hand agility problems. Some shufflers will accommodate up to three decks of cards, but unfortunately only regular-sized playing cards can be used.

Hours hang heavy when mobility is curtailed. One of the recent fads which not only passes the time but teases the mind, and exercises hands, is **Rubik's cube.** According to its promotors, it is a puzzle with "three million possible combinations."

Also good for the independent at home are electronic games, which can rekindle interest in football, baseball, hockey, soccer, and other team-related sports. These games can easily be played by one or two people. In football, for instance, a person can intercept a pass, throw a fullback for a loss, or sweep around an end for a touchdown. If just one person plays, the computer will play both offense and defense. These games not only pass the time, but challenge people to think, providing the mental stimulation that many people confined to home need.

c. CRAFTS

Sewing has long been a relaxing pastime for women, and with this in mind, aids have been developed to help those with grasp problems, eye problems, and other related disabilities.

Large-headed pins now on the market make "pinning" easier for arthritic hands. Cylinder-like holders with plastic tops, which have inside magnetic rings, will not only pick up fallen pins, but when turned or twisted, the receptacle will allow pins to fall partly out of the top, making them easy to pick up. These holders are specifically designed for paper clips, but work just as well for pins, and can be purchased at any office supply store.

Threading a needle is not easy at the best of times, and for someone with a disability, it can be an impossible task. **Needle-threaders** are available at all sewing outlets and mail order sewing departments.

A needle threader is quite a simple device. The needle is secured in a pin cushion or other solid surface. Then the threader is pushed through the needle eye, the thread is passed through the loop of the threader, and the threader is withdrawn through the needle eye.

Scissors can be difficult to hold if the person has a grasp problem. Various designs have been adapted to those needs. People who have been right-handed all their lives and, because of a stroke or arthritis, have to use their left hands can now purchase **left-handed scissors.** These simply have the blades and handles reversed.

There are other types of scissors with a flexible spring strap or loop that is connected to the handle, making them self-opening.

Sometimes **thread clippers,** which can be lightly clasped in the palm of the hand, are found to be easier to use than regular scissors. These clippers place most of the stress on the thumbs, with a spring action opening them after each cut.

Stitch-witchery is just one of the trade names for an iron-on thermoplastic webbing which eliminates the use of a needle and thread altogether. It is available at most sewing and fabric outlets.

Knee clamp holders are available for those people with limited hand use. These come with one or two attachments: one has a frame for embroidery; the other has a darning egg for mending. One device even includes a holder for knitting and crocheting.

From England comes a **knitting aid,** which is a frame to hold the needle. It clamps to a chair arm or table, allowing a person with use of only one hand to practice their craft.

The regular wooden frame opens and closes on the needle, holding it securely so that the good hand is free to knit. All sizes of needles will fit this frame.

For those with limited funds, knitting needle holders can be fashioned at home. Wing nuts make good "turners" on the jaws of any device.

Anyone who likes weaving, rug hooking, quilting, or similar frame work can purchase frames on the retail market, but these are expensive. Senior citizen workshops and drop-in centers will often make their own frames, which are just as good as the commercial ones.

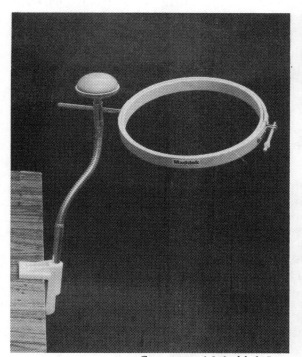

Courtesy of Maddak Inc.

Courtesy of Homecraft Supplies Limited, London, England.

Holder for knitting, crocheting, embroidery, and darning.

Knitting aid.

Homemade looms have also proven successful for those with weaving skills. First, a wooden frame is made in a rectangular shape. Ordinary nails with small heads are placed in tight rows across the head and foot of the frame. Unbreakable nylon or a similar type of thread is then stretched tautly back and forth around the nails from head to foot. When this is finished, a needle-like shuttle carrying the yarn or thread is woven between the nylon threads in, up and over, and down and under, rotating across the loom. Then, a slim wooden harness or ruler-like piece of wood is inserted between the elevated upper and lower threads, and pulled down to pack each weave tightly into place.

Although crude in looks, these homemade looms can turn out products such as placemats and scarves, with the crafts person's own individuality woven into the work. Semi-professionals as well as beginners are doing it.

Quilting frames and **rug-hooking frames** are being adapted, too, to fit the needs of those with limited use of their hands. These can be made at home by someone with a little ingenuity and time who is willing to suffer through a trial and error period until the right frame is developed.

Woodworking, leathercraft, stone-carving and **whittling** have always been favorite crafts for men. Now a "thumb-thing" sander, an aid that exercices the thumb as well as the arm, is available. It is a small post centered in a rectangular sander, with a plastic push-button dowel in the center that moves up and down with thumb pressure. The resistance range is 1 inch (2.5 cm), pressure ranges from 1 to 5 pounds (.45 to 2.3 kg), and the device holds a half sheet of sandpaper.

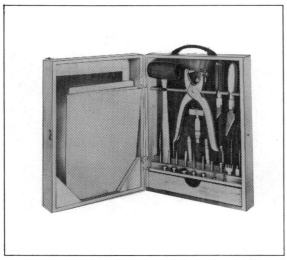

Reprinted by permission of J. A. Preston Corporation.

Leathercraft kit.

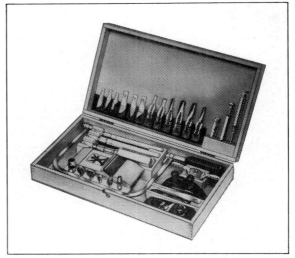

Reprinted by permission of J. A. Preston Corporation.

Woodcraft kit.

The company that manufactures thumb-thing sanders, has also devised a **super sanders set.** With this three-device set, it is possible to sand, shape or chamfer virtually any surface.

Some centers for seniors are fashioning their own devices to help people who are limited to the use of one hand, on a budget, and want to have the satisfaction of creating things.

One such contraption is a mitt-like holder secured to the hand by a velcro strap. This holder is attached to a small block of wood that has been fitted with sandpaper. The hand that is affected can be inserted into the mitt, and the good hand pushes it over the surface giving it much-needed exercise. If this is not practical, or the problem is one of grasp, either hand can be inserted in the mitt for working purposes.

There are many specially-designed **leathercraft tools** for users with limited hand use. However, they are expensive for the average person confined to home. The sets costs from $200 up. These sets, though, contain about 36 assorted tools: punches, blades, points, and an instruction manual to get the user started.

While there are also complete woodworking sets on the market, there are basic starter sets for all types of small-scale craft and hobby use.

APPENDIX

MANUFACTURERS OF AIDS

AMERICAN STAIR-GLIDE CORPORATION
4001 East 138 Street
Grandview, Missouri   64030

BELL CANADA
393 University Avenue
19th Floor
Toronto, Ontario
M5G 1W9

CANADIAN WHEELCHAIR MANUFACTURING LTD.
1360 Blundell Road
Mississauga, Ontario
L4Y 1M5

CARDON REHABILITATION PRODUCTS
3206 Wharton Way
Mississauga, Ontario
L4X 2C1

COMFORT CLOTHING KINGSTON INC.
17 Harvey Street.
Kingston, Ontario
K7K 5C1

> *Outlets:*
> Kerrisdale Equipment Ltd.
> 2095 West 41st Street
> Vancouver, B.C.
> V6M 1Y7
>
> Comfort Shop
> 4723 First Street S.W.
> Calgary, Alberta
> T2G 0A1
>
> Carefree Clothing
> 50 Academy Park Road
> Regina, Saskatchewan
> S4S 4T7

APPENDIX

> Helen Siemens
> 186 Elm Street
> Winnipeg, Manitoba
> R3M 3P2
>
> Easy Fashions
> Hampton Park Plaza
> 1381A Carling Avenue
> Ottawa, Ontario
> K1Z 7L6
>
> Community Occupational Therapy Services
> 1942 Rosebank Avenue
> Halifax, Nova Scotia
> B3H 4C7
>
> J. & P. McLelland
> P.O. Box 8745
> Station A
> St. Johns, Newfoundland
> A1B 3T2

EVEREST & JENNINGS INC.
1803 Pontius Avenue
Los Angeles, California   90025

EVEREST & JENNINGS CANADIAN LIMITED
111 Snidercroft Road
Concord, Ontario
L4K 1B6

FASHION-ABLE
Rocky Hill, New Jersey   08553

HELP YOURSELF AIDS
P.O. Box 192
Hinsdale, Illinois   60521

INDEPENDENT NEEDS CENTRE
26 Colonnade Road
Willowdale, Ontario
M2K 2L5

LUMEX INC.
100 Spence Street
Bay Shore, New York   11706

LUMEX INC.
2960 Leonis Boulevard
Los Angeles, California   90058

    In Canada:
        Medical Mart Supplies Ltd.
        1224 Dundas Street East
        Unit 28
        Mississauga, Ontario
        L4Y 4A2

MADDAK INC.
Pequannock, New Jersey   07440

NEBEL'S APPLIANCES INC.
Dolton, Illinois   60419

NOR-STAN INSTITUTIONAL PRODUCTS LTD.
491 Brimley Road
Unit 20
Scarborough, Ontario
M1J 1A4

J.T. POSEY COMPANY
5635 Peck Road
Arcadia, California   91006

J. A. PRESTON CORPORATION
60 Page Road
Clifton, New Jersey   07012

    In Canada:
        J. A. Preston of Canada Ltd.
        3220 Wharton Way
        Mississauga, Ontario
        L4X 2C1

PROTECTALERT
The Home Care Division of Extendicare Ltd.
Suite 700
1 Yonge Street
Toronto, Ontario
M5E 1S4

ROHO RESEARCH & DEVELOPMENT INC.
3105 Missouri Avenue
East St. Louis, Illinois   62205

UNITED CARE LIMITED
7 Lower Fitzwilliam Street
Dublin 1, Ireland

VOCATIONAL GUIDANCE & REHABILITATION SERVICES
2239 East 55th Street
Cleveland, Ohio   44103

WINFIELD COMPANY
46 Avenue North
St. Petersburg, Florida   33714

Other U.S. Distributors:

Abbey Medical Equipment Inc.
Catalogue Sales Department
13782 Crenshaw Boulevard
Gardena, California   90249

Whittaker General Medical Corp.
Medical Supplies & Laboratory Apparatus
8741 T Landmark Road
Richmond, Virginia   23228

Other Canada Distributors:

Doncaster Medical Ltd.
248 Steelcase Road East
Markham, Ontario
L3R 1G2

CANADIAN
ORDER FORM
SELF-COUNSEL SERIES

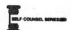

02/85

NATIONAL TITLES:	
Adopted?	3.95
Advertising for Small Business	4.95
Assertiveness for Managers	8.95
Basic Accounting	5.95
Be a Better Manager	7.95
Better Book for Getting Hired	9.95
Business Guide to Effective Speaking	6.95
Business Guide to Telephone Systems	7.95
Buying (and Selling) a Small Business	6.95
Changing Your Name in Canada	3.50
Civil Rights	8.95
Collection Techniques for the Small Business	4.95
Complete Guide to Being Your Own Home Contractor	19.95
Credit, Debt, and Bankruptcy	5.95
Criminal Procedure in Canada	12.95
Design Your Own Logo	9.95
Drinking and Driving	4.50
Editing Your Newsletter	14.95
Exporting	12.50
Family Ties That Bind	7.95
Federal Incorporation and Business Guide	12.95
Financial Control for the Small Business	5.95
Financial Freedom on $5 A Day	6.95
For Sale By Owner	4.95
Franchising in Canada	5.95
Fundraising	5.50
Getting Money	14.95
Getting Sales	14.95
Getting Started	11.95
How You Too Can Make a Million . . . In the Mail Order Business	8.95
Immigrating to Canada	12.95
Immigrating to the U.S.A.	14.95
Importing	21.95
Insuring Business Risks	3.50
Learn to Type Fast	6.50
Life Insurance for Canadians	3.50
Managing Your Office Records and Files	14.95
Media Law Handbook	6.50
Mike Grenby's Money Book	5.50
Mike Grenby's Tax Tips	6.95
Money Spinner	14.95
Mortgage and Foreclosure Handbook	5.95
Parents' Guide to Day Care	5.95
Practical Guide to Financial Management	5.95
Resort Condos	4.50
Retirement Guide for Canadians	9.95
Start and Run a Profitable Beauty Salon	14.95
Start and Run a Profitable Consulting Business	
Start and Run a Profitable Craft Business	10.95
Start and Run a Profitable Home Typing Business	9.95
Start and Run a Profitable Restaurant	10.95
Start and Run a Profitable Retail Business	11.95
Start and Run a Profitable Video Store	10.95
Starting a Successful Business in Canada	12.95
Tax Law Handbook	12.95
Taxpayer Alert!	4.95
Tax Shelters	6.95
Trusts and Trust Companies	3.95
Upper Left-Hand Corner	10.95
Using the Access to Information Act	5.95
Word Processing	8.95
Working Couples	5.50
Write Right!	(Cloth) 5.95 / (Paper) 4.95

PROVINCIAL TITLES:
Please indicate which provincial edition is required.

Consumer Book
□B.C. 7.95 □Ontario 6.95

Divorce Guide
□B.C. 10.95 □Alberta 9.95 □Ontario 9.95 □Man./Sask.

Employee/Employer Rights
□B.C. 6.95 □Alberta 6.95 □Ontario 5.50

Fight That Ticket
□B.C. 5.95 □Alberta □Ontario 3.95

Incorporation Guide
□B.C. 14.95 □Alberta 14.95 □Ontario 14.95 □Man./Sask.

Landlord/Tenant Rights
□B.C. □Alberta 5.50 □Ontario 6.95

Marriage & Family Law
□B.C. 6.95 □Alberta 5.95 □Ontario 7.95

Probate Guide
□B.C. 12.95 □Alberta 9.95 □Ontario 9.95

Real Estate Guide
□B.C. 7.95 □Alberta 4.95 □Ontario 6.50

Small Claims Court Guide
□B.C. 6.95 □Alberta □Ontario 5.95

Wills
□B.C. 5.50 □Alberta 5.95 □Ontario 5.50

Wills/Probate Procedure
□Sask./Man. 4.95

PACKAGED FORMS:

Divorce
□B.C. 12.95 □Alberta 12.95 □Ontario 14.50 □Man. 8.50 □Sask. 12.50

Incorporation
□B.C. 12.95 □Alberta 11.95 □Ontario 14.95

□Man. 7.95 □Sask. 7.95 □Federal 9.95

□Minute Books 16.50

Probate
□B.C. Administration 14.95 □B.C. Probate 14.95 □Alberta 13.95 □Ontario 15.50

Sell Your Own Home
□B.C. 4.95 □Alberta 4.95 □Ontario 4.95

□ Rental Form Kit (B.C., Alberta, Ontario, Man./Sask.)	5.95
□ Have You Made Your Will?	5.95
□ If You Love Me Put It In Writing Contract Kit	9.95
□ If You Leave Me Put It In Writing B.C. Separation Agreement Kit	14.95

NOTE: All prices subject to change without notice.

Books are available in book and department stores, or use the order form below.
Please enclose cheque or money order (plus sales tax where applicable) or give us your
MasterCard or Visa Number (please include validation and expiry date).

(PLEASE PRINT)

Name _____

Address _____

City _____

Province _____ Postal Code _____

□ Visa/ □ MasterCard Number _____

Validation Date _____ Expiry Date _____

If order is under $20.00, add $1.00 for postage and handling.

Please send orders to:

INTERNATIONAL SELF-COUNSEL PRESS LTD.   □ Check here for free catalogue.
306 West 25th Street
North Vancouver, British Columbia
V7N 2G1

AMERICAN
ORDER FORM
SELF-COUNSEL SERIES

11/84

NATIONAL TITLES

_____ Assertiveness for Managers	8.95
_____ Basic Accounting for the Small Business	5.95
_____ Be a Better Manager	7.95
_____ Business Guide to Effective Speaking	6.95
_____ Business Guide to Telephone Systems	7.95
_____ Buying (and Selling) a Small Business	6.95
_____ Collection Techniques for the Small Business	4.95
_____ Design Your Own Logo	
_____ Exporting from the U.S.A.	12.95
_____ Family Ties That Bind	7.95
_____ Financial Control for the Small Business	5.50
_____ Financial Freedom on $5 A Day	6.95
_____ Fundraising for Non-Profit Groups	5.50
_____ Franchising in the U.S.	5.95
_____ Getting Sales	14.95
_____ How You Too Can Make a Million . . . In the Mail Order Business	8.95
_____ Immigrating to Canada	12.95
_____ Immigrating to the U.S.A.	14.95
_____ Learn to Type Fast	6.50
_____ The Money Spinner	14.95
_____ Parents' Guide to Day Care	5.95
_____ Practical Guide to Financial Management	5.95
_____ Resort Condos and Time Sharing	4.50
_____ Retirement in the Pacific Northwest	4.95
_____ Start and Run a Profitable Beauty Salon	14.95
_____ Start and Run a Profitable Craft Business	10.95
_____ Start and Run a Profitable Home Typing Business	9.95
_____ Start and Run a Profitable Restaurant	10.95
_____ Start and Run a Profitable Retail Business	11.95
_____ Start and Run a Profitable Video Store	10.95
_____ Starting a Successful Business on West Coast	12.95
_____ Upper Left-Hand Corner	10.95
_____ You and the Police	3.50
_____ Word Processing	5.50
_____ Working Couples	4.50

STATE TITLES
Please indicate which state edition is required.

_____ Divorce Guide
☐ Washington (with forms) 12.95 ☐ Oregon 11.95

_____ Employee/Employer Rights
☐ Washington 5.50

_____ Incorporation and Business Guide
☐ Washington ☐ Oregon 11.95

_____ Landlord/Tenant Rights
☐ Washington 5.95 ☐ Oregon 6.95

_____ Marriage and Family Law
☐ Washington 4.50 ☐ Oregon 4.95

_____ Probate Guide
☐ Washington 9.95

_____ Real Estate Buying/Selling Guide
☐ Washington 5.95 ☐ Oregon 3.95

_____ Small Claims Court
☐ Washington 4.50

_____ Wills
☐ Washington ☐ Oregon 5.95

PACKAGED FORMS
_____ Divorce
☐ Oregon Set A (Petitioner) 12.95
☐ Oregon Set B (Co-Petitioners) 12.95

_____ If You Love Me — Put It In Writing 7.95

_____ Incorporation
☐ Washington 12.95 ☐ Oregon 10.50

_____ Probate
☐ Washington 6.50

_____ Will and Estate Planning Kit 4.95

All prices subject to change without notice.

Please send orders to:

SELF-COUNSEL PRESS INC.
1303 N. Northgate Way
Seattle, Washington 98133

☐ Check here for free catalog

(PLEASE PRINT)

NAME _____

ADDRESS _____

CITY _____

STATE _____

ZIP CODE _____

Check or Money Order enclosed ☐

If order is under $20.00, add $1.50 for postage and handling.